A WISE BIRTH

Also by Penny Armstrong and Sheryl Feldman

A Midwife's Story

A WISE BIRTH

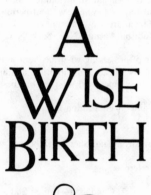

Bringing Together the Best of
Natural Childbirth with Modern Medicine

Penny Armstrong, C.N.M., and Sheryl Feldman

WILLIAM MORROW AND COMPANY, INC.
New York

Recognizing the importance of preserving what has been written, it is the policy of William Morrow and Company, Inc., and its imprints and affiliates to have the books it publishes printed on acid-free paper, and we exert our best efforts to that end.

Library of Congress Cataloging-in-Publication Data

Armstrong, Penny.
  A wise birth / Penny Armstrong and Sheryl Feldman.
    p. cm.
  Includes bibliographical references.
  ISBN 0-688-09192-X
  1. Obstetrics—United States. 2. Childbirth—United States.
I. Feldman, Sheryl. II. Title.
RG518.U5A76 1990
618.4'0973—dc20   89-48524
                                                                        CIP

Printed in the United States of America

First Edition

1 2 3 4 5 6 7 8 9 10

BOOK DESIGN BY PAUL CHEVANNES

For Anarcha

Contents

Introduction

FEW YEARS back my friend Penny Armstrong and I wrote *A Midwife's Story,*[1] a book about her experiences as a midwife for the Amish people of Pennsylvania. In that unusual setting, we observed and described births that were accomplished with very little fuss. Typically, the woman labors, and as birth approaches, she goes to her bedroom, lies on her side, and pushes her baby out. No drugs, no cuts, only a few very small tears. After attending sixty to eighty births like this myself, I had no trouble believing that birth could be a healthy, usually satisfying event in a woman's life and that women could do it pretty much on their own.

After the book came out, we received letters from women who wanted to have their next baby "Penny's way," that is, without knife and drugs. They complained about having been needled, tested, wired up, put on their backs, tied into stirrups, cut, sewn, and otherwise dismantled and deconstructed. They were bitter about having

9

had their babies taken away from them after birth so that they too could be tested, probed, cleaned out, needled, and observed. They felt that the way they had given birth may have unnecessarily compromised their bodies and the vitality of their newborns.

I knew their complaints were not specious. Approximately 60 percent of women in America today have episiotomies—surgical cuts to the perineum—when they give birth. The vast majority do receive drugs, which pass to the baby and repress respiration and circulation. An astonishing one woman in four has a cesarean section, which is major surgery and requires a relatively lengthy period of recovery.[2]

On the other hand—thanks to the education I had received from Penny—I was aware that episiotomies are occasionally required in a birth; that there are times when a woman and her baby, for complex reasons, benefit from having drugs administered during labor; and that some cesareans are unequivocally life-saving.

Nevertheless, the statistical disparity between the two groups of women was dramatic: About 1 percent of Penny's clients have episiotomies; about 6 percent end up with cesareans. It certainly didn't seem fair to me that one group of women should be able to have babies without much intervention while the other group—the one that I, in fact, most identified with—generally got cut.

What confounded me was the inconsistency between the typical hospital births, which restrict a woman, and the character of women of childbearing age. One of most striking qualities of American women today is that they are exploring and expanding their capabilities. On the job, they'll ask themselves: How efficient can I be in my work, how convincing in a speech, how objective when criticized, how energetic in selling, how patient with detail, how able with customers and clients, how organized with my resources? They are assertive, or learning to be; many of them are comfortable with power or determined to become so. In childbirth, by contrast, the majority of women behave passively, requesting drugs that will diminish not only pain, but power and effectiveness. Many have their babies taken out of them, rather than pushing them out themselves. These two behaviors—the one outward and self-discovering and the other inward and self-abnegating—appeared to be contradictory.

In discussing the problem, Penny and I ruled out the possibility that it was all the physicians' doing. If one in four women had cesareans, then women must, somehow, be in agreement with them. We felt we must be seeing a social pattern, not the raid of a group of misogynists on unsuspecting females. An explanation of birthplace habits, therefore, had to be complex and, even if unintentionally, collusive: Society in general, including birthing mothers, has legitimate, if not particularly healthy, reasons for participating in and perpetuating the highly medicalized birth.

In order to understand why women choose medicalized births, we interviewed about sixty women who were either pregnant or had recently had babies. We chose to concentrate on white, educated women. Although theirs is a miniculture and therefore not entirely representative of the population at large (indeed, the cesarean rate of well-educated, professional women is higher than the national average), we had learned from birth history that the upper classes set birth trends.

Louise de Vallière, the favorite mistress of Louis XIV, for example, is said to be the first woman to have delivered on her back, knees propped up, orifices exposed, so that her lover could peek through the drapes and see the perineal crowning of his child.[3] Queen Victoria is credited with making it acceptable for women to accept chloroform during labor.[4] In nonregal America, it was upper-class women who first replaced midwives with physicians.

We made a point of asking each woman to describe her birth, but otherwise our interviews were open-ended. We felt that if we let the women introduce topics, we would learn of the pressures and influences they felt, rather than ones we hypothesized. Undirected, women placed their births within the context of the other concerns of their lives. They talked about identity, about their mate's involvement with birth and parenting, about child care and economic necessity as they intermingled with motherhood. In other words, they explained how their birth decisions made sense for them. We continued to interview women, usually in sessions that wound down naturally after an hour and a half, until we reached a point when we realized we were hearing the same observations variously expressed.

What the women told us led us to interview midwives and obstetricians. We visited hospitals in this country and in England. We went to birth centers, sat in on childbirth educator programs, attended national and international conferences, and visited two midwifery schools. We talked to fathers, grandfathers, and grandmothers.

We found collusion. Although its sources are complex and its dynamics changing, we marked its beginning with Twilight Sleep, a drug that was introduced into the birth chamber in 1914 and used into the early sixties. Twilight Sleep was a combination drug—a mix of morphine, which subdues pain; Phenergen, an antiemetic and relaxant; and, most significantly, scopolamine, which is an amnesic. Twilight Sleep was enthusiastically embraced by physicians, who said that it was a return to a more natural form of childbirth. Under its influence, a woman labored freely and actively, rather as an animal might; she even felt pain. But because of the amnesia-inducing qualities of scopolamine, she did not remember her labor, her pain, or, for that matter, giving birth. Of particular advantage to the attending physician was that the woman under the influence of Twilight Sleep usually did as her doctor told her.

Twilight Sleep is a symbol of the loss of the birthing legacy among women. Prevented from remembering the pain of birth, women were also deprived of feeling its power. Unable to experience, personally and intimately, the resurrective, reproductive power of nature flowing through them, they came to believe that their bodies—and their characters—were insufficient to birth. Those who witnessed their helplessness, that is, their caregivers, believed the same and became ever more occupied with shoring up the birthing woman. The beliefs persist today, thoroughly institutionalized. It is so pervasive that we tend to think that a woman must be exceptional in order to engage in a natural physiological function.

We will argue, however, that in today's birth environment, women and their caregivers are correct in making this judgment. We will also argue that it is the environment, and not women's bodies, that make birth far more difficult than it need be. Ultimately, we will show that it is quite possible today for not particularly courageous women to have their babies with a vitality that abets mothering and family.

There are many voices in the book, including ours, which are the organizing ones. Sometimes Penny and I write in one voice, sometimes only for ourselves. We set it up this way because we discovered the book together and because we knew from that experience that two heads really are better than one. I'm not equipped to make authoritative statements about the intricacies of childbirth. Penny, who is a certified nurse-midwife and who has has attended more than 1200 births, the vast majority of them at home, handles these clinical complexities with grace and expertise. To her knowledge, I was able to add my training in the history of ideas and my experience of giving birth and raising two children. So we drew from both our minds and lives, letting them blend or split off as seemed appropriate. For the sake of continuity, I did the actual writing.

Sheryl Studley Feldman
with
Penny Bradbury Armstrong

ON THE POWER

My FRIEND Penny, who is a nurse-midwife, assists Amish women having babies at home, and sometimes I go out with her. I remember one woman particularly. Rachel[1] was young, unformed, and vastly uncertain. She was so shy, in fact, that she scuttled beetle-like across the open spaces of her very own kitchen, one of those Amish girls whose experience of the outside world was limited to what she heard from her more adventurous friends, ones who had, in fact, walked through a shopping mall.

Of course Rachel wanted to do her best with her birth, but she hadn't any idea of what was entailed, so we were out to her house several times on false alarms. The minute Penny cut the engine of the car, the screen door would bang and Sam, Rachel's husband, would lope out of the house to greet us. Each time, he'd lead us indoors to Rachel, who would be seated in the recesses of her couch, crocheting intently on an ever-lengthening afghan. Sam stood next

17

to her protectively. Penny would ask Rachel questions and she would answer in muffled responses, as if from the inside of her stitches.

"You were having more pains then, Rachel," Penny would say.

"There were quite a lot this morning."

"How long did they last?"

"There was one forty-five seconds, wasn't there, Sam?" she'd say.

And Penny would say, "That's good. You're doing just fine," and she would sit down beside Rachel. She used words meant for a woman with an eighth-grade education and farmyard experience. "Your body's getting some of its work done ahead of time. It's turning the soil." Penny would pick up a stretch of afghan and admire it. "You won't be getting your baby until the contractions are regular and lasting. You'll feel the difference."

Rachel would nod and hook.

"Are you drinking your red raspberry tea?" Penny would ask, referring to an herb that softens the opening of the uterus.

"We make sure to that," her boy-husband might announce. His married man's beard, only ten months in the growing, was struggling to cover his jaw.

When the final call came late on a Sunday night, the afghan was lapping around Rachel's ankles. She dropped her hook as we came into the kitchen, closed her eyes, sucked in her lower lip, and vanished into a contraction. Penny told Sam he might fit us up with some light and soon we were following a lantern into the bedroom, where Penny examined Rachel. The news was good.

"We thought maybe this time was different," Sam said, gleaming.

"We'll be needing the big red suitcase in the back of the car," Penny told him. "It'll be heavy enough for you." He set directly off.

When he brought it in, I straightened the rubber gloves, syringes, suction equipment, and suture packs. I unlatched the black box that held the oxygen tank. While I worked, Sam brought a plastic bucket to the bedroom, found the homestitched pads for spreading on the bed, threw back the covers, smoothed the sheet, and set out the pad himself. Then he went into the kitchen where, from the sounds, I knew he was balancing a cookie sheet on a kitchen scale—a make-shift device for weighing the new baby.

Rachel labored for several hours, sometimes walking, sometimes with Sam rubbing her back. After a while she took a position in the tight alley between her bed and chest of drawers, apparently buying resistance against pain by pressing her back on the bottom bureau drawer. None of us spoke much during that time. Later she got back up on the bed and not too long afterward we smelled the burst of sweat that marks the beginning of the pushing phase of labor.

She threw the force of her contractions against the bone of her pelvis. Her groans came not from her throat but from the cave parts of her body. As the baby traveled, Rachel's bones and muscles gave way. The ligaments and tendons, warmed by the vigor of labor and pressured by waves from the contracting uterus, eased out, and eventually we could make out the dark ridges on the top of the baby's head. It should have been two, three contractions before she emerged, but the baby snagged on the last notch of her mother's tailbone. For six or seven pushes, the baby rocked forward infinitesimally and retreated, but Rachel, too absorbed in her labor to notice, did not complain.

Penny guided Rachel onto her knees. "Sam," Penny said, "when the next contraction comes, I want you to push here," and she took his hand and placed it on his wife's back. Without a word, he climbed on the bed, and when the next wave came, the heel of his hand rode down with it.

Three contractions clapped down, and then the baby's head was ringed by a tight halo of Rachel's perineum. It spread and a head slid out. Penny's fingers went to the baby's neck, where she found a cord and unlooped it. We waited while the head pivoted and then there was another contraction and a baby girl, tossing us reassuring cries, was landed by her mother's knees.

Rachel, timid and tentative, authoritative about nothing more than beating mashed potatoes smooth and hanging clothes in order on the line, had borne her cord-noosed, backbone-snagged child. In the process, she experienced the power that accompanies motherhood.

There is power that comes to women when they give birth. They don't ask for it, it simply invades them. Accumulates like clouds on the horizon and passes through, carrying a child with it. Penny and I have both known it. Penny, one hand on a woman's knee, has seen it steal into a lackluster labor and radiate a child out. I felt it erupting in me when I had my children. It sounds in our bodies. Contractions creep up, seizing ever stronger until they make a mockery of all the work we have ever done on our own. Birth can silence our ego and, for the moment, we feel ourselves overcome by a larger life pounding through our own.

The experience of power is an appropriate introduction to parenthood, which also explodes in our guts. "You'll see," many of our mothers said to us when we were growing up. "Just wait until you have children of your own." And they were right, we have to wait, because we can't imagine the bolt that comes. Not only does parenthood expand our physical and psychological endurance, but it also invades every character trait we've got. So desperately do we want to make patience, generosity, tolerance, compassion, commitment, affection, common sense, courage, and humor flow that we suffer cruelly when we find our resources too small. One trouble with having children is that they reveal who we are; what makes it worse, we care. We care overwhelmingly. "The deep, deep love," a new mother and editor at *National Geographic* said. "I knew that wild animals would defend their babies. I know now that I would kill for mine." So fierce are mothers.

When you see the power flowing uninterrupted, as we did in Rachel's birth, it seems as predetermined as that mother's fierce love. As absolute, as single-minded, as disregarding of human affairs as weather. Sometimes, as an assistant, you are pulled in by it and you lose your capacity to think about it; at other times you watch it, as if through a living room window, and find yourself feeling like a child, disarmed by the universe and all the amazing forces that dwell in it. In these moments, you think it can't be stopped.

But for all its mythic force, the power is vulnerable. It can be undercut. It can and will stall, wallow, and punish. It can and will be capricious, vengeful, and sulky. It can and will retreat, grow taciturn, withold. It can take a child's life. Sometimes it seems like God in the Old Testament, giving a woman a bad time for no reason that we humans can make out. As a result, it's hard to be sanguine about birth.

So women prepare, plan, and protect themselves for nature's eventualities. They bring experts into their lives when they are with child, trusting that these people have some familiarity with the mercurial maneuvers of nature. They read, they make arrangements and informed decisions. They think how to cope with the pain. We hope to trim birth down to size, hoping that she'll behave herself in our ordinary, nonmythical lives.

Penny and I go about listening to women's birth stories. We make arrangements to talk to Leslie, a professional woman and the mother of six-month-old Nathan. It's midafternoon in an eastern city in November and we're looking chilly, so she gives us coffee and almond cookies before she starts with her story.

"You get what a friend of mine calls 'baby lust,' " she said. "My husband had it too." Not sure if it was professionally convenient for them to have baby lust, they had it anyway and got pregnant. (As luck would have it, the baby's due date coincided with the end of a major project Leslie had been working on.) They found a doctor who was "young and not paternalistic. He didn't say tummy or bottom and all that. He was very frank and open." He recommended a couple of books and Leslie and her husband, Craig, attended childbirth classes at the hospital. They thought it would be helpful to "learn their procedures." By the time the classes were completed, Leslie understood the choices she would be making during her labor and delivery. She felt that if she wanted to give birth without drugs, she could. Her question was whether she wanted to.

Cool-headed and casual, Leslie was clearly accustomed to making decisions. Her organizational skills were apparent in her home which, despite the encroachment of baby paraphernalia, was ordered. Before we left, we would be tortured by the aroma of chicken and curry, which had begun to cook itself in timely fashion.

The idea of avoiding anesthetics for the sake of "some ideal" didn't wash with her. "Sometimes," she said, breaking a cookie and popping half of it into her mouth, "you hear people obsessed with prepared childbirth say, 'The pain is good to feel.' If men said that, we'd say it was incredibly sexist."

That's for sure, we said.

Then she leaned over her cup, which meant that her magnificent black hair, cut like Cleopatra's, closed over her face and that we lost sight of her green eyes. "I had had an abortion . . . ," she said, securing her hands on her coffee cup. "It was a terrible, terrible experience. . . . With each contraction in the abortion, I had a terrific wave of nausea and at the end I was literally paralyzed . . . I couldn't open my eyes . . . I thought I was dying.

"The doctor," she proceeded, "just kept telling me it didn't hurt. . . . He screamed at me when I called him the next day." Head down, fingertips drumming, she was snapping events together efficiently, as if they had been jacket closings. "I was really afraid my labor would be the same way, that I would be paralyzed. I had no idea what caused it because the doctor wouldn't discuss it with me. . . . I thought it was emotional, that it was maybe anxiety. So I thought, if you have to take something to dull the pain to avoid that, well just do it.

"I told my obstetrician [about the paralysis] and he said, 'I won't promise you something like that won't happen, but I don't think it will.' " Her head came up then and her eyes rejoined us.

With the ambivalence about her body in her mind, she carried her baby to term and went into labor near her due date. "People had described labor contractions as like an earthquake wracking your whole body. It was totally unlike that. It was all very, very contained like in this little belt," she said, adding that she'd sustained herself by sitting on the hospital bed and resting her head on her husband's shoulder. When nausea hit, "I said to myself, you can take something and you don't have to feel this pain anymore." She spoke to the nurse, who offered an epidural, to numb the lower body, but the doctor ordered Demerol, an analgesic. They may have gotten her on her back then, cinched the strap of the fetal monitor[2] around her belly, and switched the monitor on.

With the Demerol in her veins, Leslie fell into a sludgy sleep. "I didn't want to breathe," she said. "My husband tried to wake me to tell me to breathe. I said, 'Why should I breathe when I can sleep?' " While she slumbered, her body labored on, and when it came time to push the doctor insisted that she come to.

Unenthusiastic about being awake, not feeling the drive to push, she pushed for two hours, and then the baby banked on her tailbone, its heartbeat dropped, the doctor cut an episiotomy and pulled the baby out with forceps. The cord, he said, had been around the baby's neck. "It took them about a minute to get him to breathe, but Nathan was fine."

"Anyway," she said, casually dropping her lush head to her hand, "it took the doctor and the resident forty minutes to stitch up the episiotomy."

"Forty?" one of us gasped.

She nodded and went on to say that her mouth had been dry as sand and her legs quivering the whole time they stitched. She must have seen us shaking our heads, because she tackled us with a cynical remark. "You know how after the baby's delivered everybody forgets about you."

"Uhmm," we said.

While she was in the hospital, she went on to say, she had a "kind of distant feeling" toward Nathan. It was "nice" to nurse him, but she felt no extraordinary surge of emotion; besides, her mouth was incredibly dry and all she could think of was drinking water. She brought Nathan home and for the first day was in a daze. On the second day she went to check on him while he slept and, hovering over the rail of the crib, she fell helplessly in love with him. Seeing him from this new perspective, she began to attack herself for giving him a stressful birth.

We went on talking after that, about Leslie's career plans, her baby-sitting problems, and the mothering decisions she was faced with, but as soon as Penny and I hit the sidewalk, the first words out of our mouths were something like: Darn right it was stressful. Stressful for the baby who got hung up in the birth canal, who had to be dragged out by forceps, who had to be poked and prodded to breathe. Stressful for Leslie, who literally toughed her way through, past perceived inadequacies, into and out of complex decisions, pushed when her body wanted to sleep, and ended up cut. What's more, she'd done it without the accompaniment of much power. Slovenly thing, it did not appear and wash Nathan out into the doctors' hands. It left Leslie to muscle the child out, as if she were an athlete in a competition. As if life can come about without the assistance of nature.

But Leslie, who had reported so many terrible experiences to us so matter-of-factly, had made but one bitter comment: ". . . everybody forgets about you." Sitting on the bus, we returned to those words. It was true, we said, they had. Amidst doctors, nurses, childbirth educators, hospital staff, sensitive machinery, sophisticated knowledge, all focused on successful outcome, the woman with the black hair and the baby lust, the human in whom life had re-created itself, had been ignored.

Not just at the end, although that's what she said, but all the way through. There was the abortionist who concealed information from her; the doctor who gave her casual comfort when she was worrying about whether her body, her baby's life source, might not sabotage her and him; the nurse who failed to explain to her that a bolt of nausea meant not paralysis, but a vigorous and active labor; the books that did not tell her that her baby would travel better on her undrugged strength; the people who, apparently afraid that she might move as women move—wide-hipped, rhythmic, and yielding—had made her hips lie still, straight, and narrow on a hard table, no place for making love or giving birth.

We knew Leslie's birth was not exceptional. Indeed, among the women we talked to and in the society at large, such births are typical. Each woman may be an individual, each birth may be different, but what is constant is the supplanting of the formidable undulation of muscles, hormones, and bones by needles, wires, tubes, chemicals, and metal objects. What is routine is the diminution of power. What is common is the absence of respect. What lasts is the sense of failure.

Out of instinct and desire, we make children. Dependent on the genius of our bodies, we grow them in our wombs. If and when we defer to that same genius during birth, if and when we invite and cultivate its power, we find that women can give birth 85 to 90 percent of the time without complication and without unreasonable bravery. Seeing birth work well, seeing that women generously attended abide its pain and rejoice in its fruition, we remember that nature wants her young. We find that the power that comes to woman at birth is not, after all, as inconstant as it might seem. It can be derailed, diminished, even paralyzed, but that's often our doing. It is like the women who carry it, becoming silent only when it is not respected. It is most painful when it is not understood.

We ignore the power foolishly, for the knowledge of nature wanting her young is our ally in birth. Not only does it carry our children out, but it follows us into our work as parents, which is formidable. It is we, after all, who must protect our babies while they are so desperately vulnerable. We who must root and ground them as they grow. We who must see their gifts and nourish them. We who must teach them to believe in themselves even when they experience failure. We who must love them enough so that they can endure hate. We who must make them thrive.

Given the responsibilities of the mother, it is odd that we cripple the power that comes with birth. It is curious that we do not give human warmth, which attenuates pain. It is strange that we mute a woman's physical and emotional responses when, well nurtured, they can give her strength. It is unthinkable that we, wanting human life to go on, cut, wound, sap, and scar the women who do the work for us.

Yet we employ these procedures routinely, regularly, even ritualistically. And send women like Leslie home to work out how it came to be. What is wrong with her that her body had to be cut, she must wonder. Why wasn't she very interested in her baby those first couple of days, she must ask. Does every woman resent the slowly healing wounds on which she sits while learning to nurse? Leslie stands alone over the baby's crib and faults herself for her baby's birth stress.

She does not accuse us—those of us who failed to be generous to her, to name her strengths, to nourish her, to give to her, to support her in the huge piece of work she is undertaking for herself, for her child, and ultimately for humankind. She does not notice the absence of humility, awe, and caring among us; instead, she absorbs the neglect, the nonanswers, the damage, and the responsibility. She criticizes herself. She suspects that her child has been hurt and she grieves. She lives with the memory of the experience and the judgment she makes of herself as a mother for the rest of her life.

PART I

THE NATURE OF BIRTH

Introduction

IN THE first chapter we contrasted the hospital birth of Leslie, a well-educated urban woman, to the home birth of Rachel, a woman who knew how to keep a farm kitchen. One can argue that the comparison is specious, the women's lives and cultures being so different. Or complain about it. Incantations about lovely, natural births tend to call up outdated images from the sixties or suggest a holier-than-thou mentality. Worse, they can cause guilt: They suggest that today's women, who already have overwhelming work and home responsibilities, should also be second-guessing their physicians, challenging state-of-the-art medicine, assuming the unknowns (for them) of home birth, and withstanding pain for the sake, as Leslie so aptly put it, "of some ideal." American women are getting their babies and Leslie and her son are hardly doomed.

In interviewing women, we quickly learned that the truly natural birth—that is, the one without drugs and technological interventions—was not attractive. Since these were well-educated, highly responsible women, we knew that their opinion of natural birth was not an unexamined one. These were women who chose to have children, who understood (as much as that is possible before the fact) the responsibility they were taking on, and who wanted to do the best they could for themselves and their children. Considering their personal qualities, we had to conclude that the natural birth was not serving them well.

Our question was, why not? If it was not a matter of character—non-Amish women toughed their way through difficulties as much as, if not more than, Amish women did—neither was it a question of information: For two decades, the benefits of the unmedicated birth have been advertised. Since that message has been rejected, one must assume that it misses something significant in the realities of childbearing today. Women have good reasons for giving birth as they do.

Penny and I, sitting in her living room, home from yet another lovely birth, reckoned with the problem. Why would the natural birth work for Amish women and fail other women? Why does that power flood rural bedrooms and dry up in hospitals? Most important, why should Penny's client population routinely enjoy outcomes that are dramatically superior to those of other women?

Penny has assisted more than twelve hundred births. At home, she uses no analgesics or regional anesthetics because they can repress infant respiration; nationally, the rate of use of epidurals (a regional anesthetic) is 60 percent. Her episiotomy rate is less than 1 percent; the national rate is 61 percent. Her transfers to physician and/or hospital care are less than 10 percent. Cesareans (which she, of course, does not do and which are included in the transfer rate) represent 6 percent; the national figure is 24 percent. Her perinatal mortality rate—which includes stillbirths and infant deaths in the first seven days of life—is 5 per thousand; nationally the figure is 10.4 per thousand (1986).[1]

Penny's an excellent practitioner. Furthermore, she's developed some skills that are unique in the birthplace today. She is the first to say, however, that clinical expertise cannot account for the disparity between her statistics and national ones. If her skills then, are not the controlling factor in outcome; if we reject as absurd the idea that non-Amish women are intrinsically lesser birthers than Amish women, we are forced back to the objection we began with: Birth may be as much a product of culture as it is of physiology.

If that is so, then the next question was whether it was possible to identify those factors that benefited birth in one culture and transfer them to another. Our opportunity, we realized, was to think of the Amish as a naturally occurring control group, a laboratory, a tool for understanding how culture infiltrates the physiologic process of birth. By comparing and contrasting Amish and mainstream experience, we might be able to get down to the generic cultural factors that favored birth. If we could do that, then we could see if they were or were not transferable. If they were transferable, then mainstream women might be able to have births from which they did not have to heal.

Ultimately we considered the effects of place on birth, we examined the traditions of medical science, we looked at what women learned from their mothers about birth and mothering, we compared the way doctors and midwives perceived and managed birth, we reexamined the information birth reformers and educators have been providing, we considered the influence of men in the birthplace and in parenting, and we tried to understand how women's other responsibilities affected their births. By these inquiries, we were able to see how to transpose the benefits of one culture to another.

We didn't begin the project until Penny had put in eight years as a midwife and the same eight taking apart the education she'd acquired during her training as a certified nurse-midwife (CNM).[2] Her education had not adequately accounted for the births she saw in farmhouses and she was obliged to develop a revised definition of the nature of birth. In the sections that follow, she describes what she found and how she came to explain it.

The Nature of Power

I'VE EXPLAINED elsewhere how I ended up doing home births for the Amish people of Lancaster County[1] and will only repeat what seems necessary here. I took my midwifery training in Scotland and at Booth Maternity Hospital in Philadelphia. I had just gotten my accreditation as a certified nurse-midwife when I responded to a call from a general practitioner out in agricultural Lancaster County, Pennsylvania. He was interested in expanding his practice among the Amish people and wanted a midwife as part of his service team. I had been raised in the country and it appealed to me to return.

When I went out for the interview, I was disturbed to find that I would be expected to do home births. All my experience with birth had been in the hospital and I was keen on having emergency equipment nearby and doctors available. I wondered if the doctor wasn't being a bit cavalier about his Amish clients. They had only eighth-grade educations, they did not sue, and so could easily be taken advantage of.

But he took me around to chat with some of the women in their homes and they told me in their own words that they preferred to have their babies at home because it was economical and it suited their farm- and family-centered, low-tech lives. Until recently, Dr. Grace Kaiser[2] had assisted them at home, but she had retired, and they were forced to choose between the hospital or one other home birth practitioner—a person whose methods, when I heard about them, I couldn't condone. What the couples said convinced me that one didn't force mainstream standards—that is, everyone goes to the hospital—on the Amish. I accepted the job and its requirement of attending home births.

I was a well-prepared midwife, exacting of myself and, in one way, ambitious. I was determined that the women I cared for would have the safest, best births possible. I immediately assessed the realities of home birth—being alone in the middle of the night at an Amish farm with my work area lit by gaslight and the closest phone a five- or ten-minute walk away—and compensated. I bought a two-way radio. I equipped the suitcase that Sheryl mentioned in the first chapter with all the drugs that midwives are licensed to carry. I put in Pitocin for the resistant placenta, Methergine for postpartum bleeding, Valium to counteract a suddenly elevating blood pressure, Epinephrine to compensate for the sometimes ill effects of numbing drugs used for episiotomy, pills for severe afterpains, antibiotics for the person at risk of infection. I put in Amni-hooks (plastic instruments for breaking the bag of waters), syringes, intravenous (IV) fluids, a ring forceps for examining the cervix, a variety of clamps and scissors, a suture kit, needles, a DeLee's suction catheter for clearing the baby's air passageway, a heavy oxygen tank, a laryngoscope for viewing the baby's throat, an endotracheal (ET) tube to slip down its airway to get oxygen to the lungs, and a bag for forcing oxygen into the baby's lungs.

The doctor and I eliminated (we call it risking out) those women whom we thought unsuitable for home birth. No mothers whose babies were in an odd position, no mothers having their tenth child (or more), no twins, no women with high blood pressure, no women with severe medical problems, no small-bodied women who seemed to be carrying big babies. Any known chance of a complication sent a woman to the hospital.

Meanwhile, I began attending births at home. I hadn't made many forays before I realized that I was seeing births for which I had not been prepared. Accustomed as I was to the taut, often breathless birth atmosphere of hospital births, I was struck by the casual, comfortable movements of the women laboring in their kitchen and giving birth among quilts. Having based much of my assessment of myself as a practitioner on my ability to respond swiftly and accurately to emergency situations, I was undone by the infrequency of the need for me to display my masterly strokes. Birth appeared to be another animal out in the country. Labors were shorter than I was accustomed to. Pain appeared to be less severe. Cuts and tears fewer. Hemorrhage controllable. Babies did not need my suctioning devices or my tubes pressed down their throats; they gurgled when they were born and began to breathe. Their mothers took them to their breasts and nursed without much complication. If problems did arise anytime during a birth, most of them appeared to resolve themselves in short order.

I had an eerie sense of unreality. The births had not only power, but grace and simplicity. Coming home at four or five in the morning after births, each one seeming to unwind to a fruitful, healthy end, I groped for explanation. I wondered if I was witnessing a statistically aberrant population of women, ones who were, by genetic predisposition, good birthers. At other times, bewitched by the grace of the starry landscape and disarmed by the humility of the Amish, I indulged in the magical idea that God rewarded people who followed a religious way of life by giving them easier births. By daylight, the clinician in me credited the food the women ate, the number of hours they spent squatting in the garden, the herbs they took, and their experience with animals giving birth. Sometimes, when sleep-deprived, I considered the self-serving possibility that it was me making all the difference. Finally I countenanced the possibility that I had stumbled upon—as I vaguely put it—something extraordinary.

I yearned to have a more experienced professional explain to me what was going on but I was reluctant to discuss my statistics, which were becoming astounding, with my mentors back at Booth. Once

I mumbled something about them and it was suggested that I wait for the other shoe to drop. That sounded like good advice, so I kept my mouth shut and maintained my style of attending women. I kept the hospital ways I had been able to bring with me into homes. I stayed with the women through the early parts of their labor, I scrubbed carefully, I watched the clock, I shone a strong flashlight on the perineum while I worked, I recorded elaborate detail on charts.

One August night, I was led yet another time by a typical Amish husband into a typical Amish bedroom. Silla, the mother, was propped up in her bed in a moonlit room calmly awaiting my arrival. She smiled, and then, conspiratorially, placed her index finger to her lips. She beckoned me to her side, pulled my head down so my ear was next to her mouth, and whispered. Would it suit me, she wanted to know, to leave the lamp unlit and to talk quietly? Her two-year-old, Joseph, was asleep in the corner of the bedroom and she didn't want to wake him.

My first reaction was to disabuse her of her easygoing confidence by lecturing her on the disasters that can accompany birth: how babies' lives had been saved because practitioners had picked up a tint in the amniotic fluid (waters), because they had been able to use their scissors precisely, because they were able to see when the color of a baby's face shifted. But while I was preparing this speech, my eyes followed Silla's over to damp, tousled Joseph, sleeping in his crib as contented as a puddle after a summer rain; I glanced at Silla's husband, who had competently assisted me at Joseph's birth, and I realized what was bothering me. If I assisted Silla as she requested I would be admitting that birth probably could be trusted.

My decision to do so was based on a number of considerations. I knew, for example, that Silla had had four births, each of them manifestly uncomplicated. This pregnancy had proceeded in perfect order. I knew that she was a responsible person, one who would not cling to her request for quiet and darkness if circumstances changed. I knew Joseph could flare up a lantern in an instant. I acknowledged that Joseph and Silla had a mature and subtle religious faith, one that embraced, as God's will, the unpredictable turnings of nature. I decided, in other words, to trust the accumulation of my experience among the Amish and the judgments that followed from it.

I held the flaps on the locks of my medical case so they wouldn't click; I stepped out into the kitchen to tear open the packages of rubber gloves; I laid my flashlight on the doily on the bureau so it wouldn't startle; I used my stethoscope instead of a doptone (which throws the sound of the baby's heartbeat around the room); I heard the bedsprings creak when Silla's husband climbed onto the bed beside her. Within the half-hour, I felt the slippery dome of a baby's head filling my palm and their little girl eased out. I slid her onto the mounded landscape of her mother's abdomen.

I reached over toward her and saw that she was breathing, that her eyes were open, that they were avidly exploring the bedroom around her. She was as alert and as clear-sighted as a person who has just risen out of deep meditation. When a smile slipped across her face, her perfection skimmed through me. She had come up as effortlessly and as reassuringly as the sun.

I had never seen a smile on the face of a child at birth; indeed, I'd never heard of such a thing. And even supposing, as I did later, that it was just a look of contentment I'd seen, the impact remained the same. If birth could be as easy for a mother as it was for Silla and as comfortable as it apparently was for her baby, then I needed to be able to explain why and how. Urged along by that confounding child, I began to think systematically about the causes of power and grace.

Clinical Factors

I knew that my clients' births were favorably influenced by the women's general good health. They scrub floors on their hands and knees, sling baskets of wet wash about, climb stairs, work out in the fields, and squat in their gardens. The air they breathe is relatively unpolluted. They don't drink or smoke and, while their diets are not ideal, they are quite adequate. Also, their bodies are not assaulted every day by the psychological stresses of urban life. These are such important physical advantages that, in theory, they should have served the women equally well no matter where they gave birth.

The theory, however, held up no further than the local hospital where, I knew from experience, the general population of Amish women had more difficulties than those who gave birth at home. There seemed to be several possible explanations for this phenomenon: It was something that doctors, who practiced in hospitals, did at delivery; it was something that midwives, when they practiced in hospitals, did at delivery; it was the hospital environment itself; or it was some combination thereof.

As I considered the first possibility, the doctor-assisted hospital delivery, I recalled the description one Amish woman had given me of her first birth. Mary seemed to be a good case for analysis because she's a serene person, one unlikely to exaggerate problems. Furthermore, unusual in an Amish person, she's quite well read. Instead of marrying at twenty or twenty-one as so many do, she taught in an Amish school for eight to ten years before she met Jonas, also a schoolteacher, and they married.

Pregnant with their first child, they asked around and found a physician who was reputed to be both kind and informative. They went to the library and got out books on painless childbirth, which they read at night, sitting at the kitchen table. Attending classes on how to have a baby naturally, they learned that shaves and enemas were outmoded and that lying on one's back during labor was "the worst."

"Apparently," she said, telling me about her first labor, "the hospital staff and my doctor . . . hadn't been informed [about the innovations in childbirth]. No one had told me I needed to lie on my back so the nurse in attendance could watch my contractions on the screen." With typical Amish humility, she added, "But who was I to inconvenience the nurse"—who was constantly checking her and adjusting the "cold" monitor on her stomach "which made the contractions seem worse."

She, a woman accustomed to backbreaking farmwork, found the pain "well-nigh unbearable. . . . With each contraction I felt as though a nerve was being pinched in the vagina. I wanted to scream but dared not, fearing I would lose all control." Entreating God to keep her from screaming, finding her praying capacity weak, she turned to Jonas and asked him to pray for her. He did, but told her later he thought she was contemplating death. "It was unthinkable," she said, describing the retreat of her dream of having a houseful of children, "that there'd be another time."

When she was ready to push, the nurse said that the doctor had not yet arrived and that she should pant through her contractions. In the meantime, while she panted, they moved her from bed to stretcher and from stretcher to delivery table. "The doctor breezed in cool as a cucumber" just as a contraction rose and she moaned.

" 'Don't you start screaming!' [he said].

"His abrupt tone of voice was not lost on me.

" 'Slide over,' came the next command.

"Apparently I wasn't dead center on the table.

"Flat on my back, feet in stirrups, sheet hiding the lower part of my body, the doctor, and some of his gazing companions, I gave birth to a son. I heard his cry. I thought he was mine. I wanted him on my stomach and at my breast."

She wanted to hold him, the first-born child of a long-awaited family-to-be and she wanted him for the sake of her body, she said, remembering her reading and that his suckling at her breast would contract her uterus naturally and force the placenta out. Instead, empty-armed, she felt a shot of Pitocin, the contraction-stimulating drug, stinging her thigh. Only after they extracted the placenta did they give her the baby. He was "blanketed, blond, wide-eyed" and "I laughed for the joy of him."

She wasn't allowed to keep him, however, because the episiotomy gaped. They took the baby away; she began to shiver and begged for a blanket, which they brought: a "nice skinny" one, "suitable for a July night." The doctor began a long sew. It went "on and on. I hadn't known this doctor to be a seamstress or a tailor. . . . I was no longer numb . . . I'd feel him sewing." The pain from the stitches kept her from sitting for a week.

"So much," she said cynically, "for the most lauded event of a woman's life. I cried until I couldn't cry anymore."

The nurses, by contrast, called it a "lovely" birth. And for them, encountering this quiet, loving, and well-educated couple, it probably was. One becomes accustomed to routines—including cutting of the flesh—and can get in the habit of not questioning their necessity.

But if you are not accustomed to it, it is shocking to see vibrant muscle cut. I think of muscles as being strung out on our bones like strings on a cello—vibrating with potential, as if for an extended concert. I dream about a batter with his shirt off and the graceful cresting of power that curves up from the small of his back, across his shoulders, and down his arms. To interrupt that progression of movement is an esthetic crime, and I feel sure we wouldn't do it if it were avoidable.

If a ballplayer was on a table in the operating room and if there was no other remedy but surgery, the prospect of cutting his muscles would still be sobering. Seeing him prepped and draped, we would know that everything possible had been done. Physical therapists with their baths, exercises, and massages would have exhausted their repertoire, specialists with slings and elastic bandages would have signed off. Only then would they resort to the knife.

Maybe we don't think of these women's muscles with the same regard because of where they are located. We don't see them crossing and gliding as they make our hips swing; we don't watch them spreading into broad ribbony bands when we squat down. We don't imagine them roiling with sex. Because we can't see them, maybe we think of them as static, a crude vessel fit only for containing entrails, bowels, and other oozy organs. Maybe that's what makes them easier to cut.

But I have seen the muscles in women. In the delivery room, when the cut was made across three or four major muscle groups, I've seen them retreat and lie there, shrunk back into themselves, and I felt the same way I would if a ballplayer's muscles had been cut. The same way I feel when a cellist's string snaps during a concert. The music of the body, the resonance and the potential for rapture are interrupted.

Replaying Mary's unwieldy birth advanced me only a little in my effort to analyze the benefits of home birth. As many practitioners today would admit, there was too much wrong. The back-lying labor, the cold monitor, the painful vaginal "checks," the waiting to push, the moves from bed to stretcher to delivery table, the strapping

down, the stirrups, the harshness of the doctor's orders, the withhold-
ing of the baby, the neglected postbirth chill, the shot, and the long
sew—all of these seemingly insignificant, routine factors are known
to increase anxiety and exacerbate pain. Even a nonlaboring person
would find them awkward, uncomfortable, and inhibiting. It would
be almost impossible for a birth to flow—as Silla's did—in such
circumstances.

I considered the second possible variation in the hospital delivery.
What about the perfectly healthy Amish woman who had her baby
in the hospital with a midwife's care? Would her birth be compromised simply by being in the hospital? Was a healthy birth dependent
upon the environment in which it took place?

The majority of women I attended in the hospital were having
their first babies—"primips," we call them. Primip births are challenging for several reasons. In the first place, the women don't have
any personal experience of birth. They are likely to be frightened or
anxious, which works against relaxation, which works against easy
birth. Second, their muscles are tight, and the baby has to travel
against their resistance. Their hormonal systems, too, are inex-
perienced at birth and may be slow to blend. These psychological and
physiological factors combine and create the major challenge of a
primip birth: the long labor. As a midwife attending a first-time
birther, I had a major interest in preserving a woman's energy so that
she would have enough strength left at the end to push the baby out.

I managed hospital births differently than most of the doctors did.
I told the women they could labor in any position they found comfortable, I did very few vaginal checks, I encouraged them to walk
the halls and inhabit the showers at will, I spoke to them kindly,
chatted with them about their families and farms, I said they could
give birth on their sides, half-sitting, or squatting. Even with these
advantages, however, the results were disappointing. While a good
proportion of the primips delivered without intervention, there were
several who should have, but couldn't. They would dilate fully, but
ultimately needed forceps or a section to give birth.

I knew energy loss was a major problem. The hospital, assessing
a set of complicated risk factors, had decided it was prudent to tell
women not to eat once they were in labor. While I disagreed with
their analysis of the risks, I respected it.[3] Thus the women, doing

hard physical work, ran out of energy before it was time for them to push.

There were other factors too, things that felt wrong but defied clinical analysis. In comparison to the home births I attended, hospital births were awkward. They were out of sync with Amish life. I'd tried to ease the transition: I often picked primips up at home and drove them to the hospital. I always guarded their rooms, trying to protect them from the invasion of strangers who spoke a language, bureaucratic and medical, that they couldn't understand; against fluorescent light, which they, being accustomed to lantern lighting, found painful; and against the uncommon, for them, sounds of machinery and phones. Obviously, I could only be partially successful.

What felt more damaging was the distrustful atmosphere of the hospital staff. Laboring women could not be helped by nurses who, not approving of my tolerance for a prolonged first stage (the prepushing part), would say disdainfully, "Is she still in labor?" or "Hasn't that girl delivered yet?" A woman in labor hears the doubt and loses confidence. Also, by similar but less direct means, the clinical review committee (it sets hospital policy) influenced the labors. They measured the time women were in labor against a table called the "Friedman labor curve." Designed to *de*scribe the average length of labor, many practitioners and the review committee used it the other way around—to *pre*scribe how long a labor might be. One either began pushing after twelve hours of active labor or one was a candidate for intervention. When the committee reviewed my labor records—which showed my tolerance for individual variation—they expressed unease. Although my outcomes were excellent by any hospital standards, the women I attended were not following the prescribed pattern.

That wasn't all. The administration expected women to give birth on a delivery table and my birthing room with its mattress and box springs did not conform; neither did my informal style. In time, their discomfort sprung up in me as anxiety and I'm sure I passed that feeling on to the laboring women. Perhaps I encouraged them too much, perhaps I implied urgency, perhaps they began to push before they were quite ready and so, in spite of their wholesome advantage, they failed.

Inviting Power

That's as far as I could get, analytically, in the months following Silla's birth. Having identified factors that seemed to interfere with women's progress in labor, I still could not understand why they interfered. Why should women feel more pain, as they seemed to, because they were in a hospital? Why would labor slow because a nurse expressed distrust or because I put subtle pressure on a woman? Why did the process *feel* so much easier at home? What were the physiological explanations?

About that time, I attended a conference on "Innovations in Perinatal Care: Assessing Benefits and Risks" at which Michel Odent, a French physician, was speaking on "The Undisturbed Birth." I confess that I took one look at him and prepared to leave. I couldn't imagine how this silver-haired, svelte-looking, urbane man could have anything to say that would throw light on my experiences back in the barn-ripe farmyards of Lancaster County. But Odent, bless his French charm, seduced me by the way he said "bebe" and I stayed long enough to discover his lack of arrogance. He said, for example, that he would save some time so that we—he and the audience—could "just talk," which is the sort of gossipy remark that one hears in some midwives' presentations but which was unique, as far as I knew, in physicians'. He went on to say that he was a surgeon by training and had his first experiences as a doctor on the battlefield. Some time later, he went to Pithiviers, a small town south of Paris, where he was surgical chief. Finding himself overworked, he became interested in avoiding unnecessary surgery. He noted that he did not have, at the time, any special sympathy for the laboring woman or the "bebe," nor was he enamored of birth reform. His interest was in exploring the possibility that his medical management techniques—time and patience, sparing intervention—might be as effective in birth as they were with other potential surgical problems. If so, the number of cesarean sections he was called upon to perform would be reduced.

Odent credited the midwives he worked with at Pithiviers. When he arrived, he said, they were doing the majority of deliveries, so he was able to observe the salubrious effects of their nontechnocratic methods—which contrasted markedly with those he had seen during a short stint in the obstetrics unit of a large Parisian hospital. If they were one asset in helping him make his discoveries about the "undisturbed birth," the fact that he hadn't been trained as an obstetrician was a second: He didn't have to dismantle any preconceived notions.

We could infer Odent's gifts. He had boundless curiosity, an excellent creative mind, superb capacities for observation, a knowledge of medicine and physiology, an appreciation of women, and, as I have grown to appreciate in him, an unusual enthusiasm for life. An acquaintance of mine, for example, had her baby with Odent at Pithiviers about five years ago. While she was pregnant, she was living in a seacoast town in France, where she loved bathing in the ocean, but was concerned with the effect of the cold water on her fetus. She asked Odent if her swims were advisable. "In your pregnancy," he said, revealing his confidence, "you should do what gives you pleasure."

The circumstances at Pithiviers combined with Odent's talents and led to a reformation of birth there. At each intervention—from the breaking of the waters to the cutting of the cord—the team asked themselves: Why are we doing this? What do we gain, if anything, by altering the natural process? What happens if we let labor run its own course? Thus they systematically let go of interventions. They gave up epidurals, which depressed the pushing reflex. They didn't break the bag of waters, which protected the baby's head and helped expand the opening of the uterus. They didn't cut the cord right after birth: Its last pulses brought added rich stores to the baby and, at the same time, helped to shrink the placenta so it could peel more easily from the uterine wall.

Following a logical progression, they built a new birthing room. Small, dimmed quiet, and earthtoned, its furnishings were singularly nondirective. A large mattress, with no norths or souths to it, was put on a platform in the corner, pillows thrown loosely about it. In an adjoining room, painted in lily-pond colors, they installed a pool, which women sought to labor in. During the same period at Pithiviers, attitudes toward childbirth preparation evolved. Instead of teaching women how to give birth, they merely tried to make them feel at home in the hospital. Odent invited them to weekly gather-ings. He replaced the customary lectures and films with singing and dancing and he, the midwives, nurses, pregnant men and women, new mothers, grandmothers, and fathers gave themselves pleasure. People made friends. Experienced mothers passed on tips to inex-perienced ones; grandmothers gave up their anxieties about this unusual place and its way of birth. When women did ask for labor and birth advice, Odent chatted with them—he's very good at mak-ing a woman feel as if she's the only person in the world—saying that there was no one way to give birth. The woman's body leads her and she need only follow it. The midwives and doctors would worry, if need be.

Thus women choreographed their own births: Cawing, mewing, pacing, curling around themselves, or springing their pain free, un-touched unless they asked for it. Their partners joined them, holding them, swinging them, massaging them, embracing them or not, whatever the woman wanted. Odent himself, extraordinarily sensi-tive to the privacy of the woman's encounter with her body, hung to the perimeters of the room, moving in only when needed. The women, supported by their husbands' arms, often gave birth in a semisquat.

Observing these births, Odent concluded that birth goes best if it takes place in a small, dimmed quiet, well-protected room. Indeed, he commented, if the one birthing room was not available, the women often dragged a pillow and blanket to a corner of the room where the sings were held. They would establish themselves behind the grand piano and labor in that small, secure, familiar, shadowed place.

Birth goes best if it is not intruded upon by strange people and strange events. It goes best when a woman feels safe enough and free enough to abandon herself to the process, to surrender, to go to, as Odent said, "another planet." It goes best when it is "undisturbed."

And I thought of pulling into a dark driveway and being ushered into the silence of a house quilted in night. We were undisturbed; the children were put away; the grandparents, experienced in patience and silence, were in a house nearby. We labored in lamplight, we spoke little; we were not strangers, and birth worked.

I thought of Abigail, my cocker spaniel, who had started into labor before visitors came tromping in, stopped then, and didn't start up until they left and I had locked the back door, turned off the music, and curled myself up in a rocking chair to read. I remembered that no matter how long we waited by sheep pens in my youth, there were no lambs until we turned our attention away.

Odent and I, half a world apart, he urban and me rural, had come to the same conclusions. The significant and (for me) celebratory difference between us was that he knew why the undisturbed birth worked and I didn't.

In physiological language, he said, we were talking about a "fetus ejection reflex,"[4] i.e, a spontaneous, natural process, like breathing, blinking our eyes, or having a bowel movement. As such, it is best managed not by our thinking mind, the neocortex, but by the body brain, the hypothalamus, which directs the interplay of hormones. The hypothalamic activities are most efficient when their processes are not impeded.

The easiest birth comes, therefore, when the spontaneous process is not under the laboring woman's scrutiny; that is, when a woman can leave off neocortical consciousness—thinking, analyzing, monitoring her environment, modifying her behavior for social purposes, or making decisions. If her birth environment is free from intellectual demands and control requirements, her labor will tend to be more powerful and effective. If the environment is designed to accommodate hypothalmic dominance—as low lights and minimum intrusions do—it will go more smoothly.

In one of his books, Birth Reborn, Odent mentions the difficulty he has in urging respect for the instinctual processes of the hypothalamus. " 'Instinct' . . . resonates with moralistic overtones," he writes. "[It] is often unfavorably contrasted with reason." But, he explains, asking us to reverse our usual standards of what is intelligent and what not, in birth it is most reasonable to give oneself over to one's body. "As women in labor move and act according to their instincts, they are in fact behaving extremely rationally."[5] I understood him to be saying that hormones have a logic that, unmonitored by us, is well patterned and notably trustworthy. Therefore, the most intelligent neocortical decision that one can make is to delegate responsibility for birth to hypothalmic intelligence.

The free-flowing hormonal run that follows such a decision is cyclical, intracyclical, co-cyclical, and countercyclical. From a scientific point of view, it is distressingly complex and thus not well understood (which helps explain why everyone doesn't speak as Odent does). We know enough about it, however, to begin to understand how it behaves during labor and, from that, how we can complement it during birth.

The hypothalamus makes and stores oxytocin, which is released (the trigger mechanism is not understood) by the pituitary gland. Oxytocin causes uterine contractions, which find a rhythm and increase in strength. With the pain of the contraction (uterine muscles cry out like any muscle when exerted) come endorphins, which both diminish pain and make us feel good—like after a good run or sex. (They also flow when breast milk does—a stroke of genius.) Endorphins are the allies of the laboring woman. They're in a highly responsive conversation with the pain, becoming more powerful as the contractions become stronger.[6]

While security, warmth, quiet, and darkness encourage the flow of endorphins, fear and its relative, stress, can inhibit them. Like a laboring animal in a cave, Odent said in another lecture, the female seeks a protected environment in which to give birth, so that she and her young will be in darkness and warmth, safe from predators. If she is undisturbed, she delivers; if, however, a predator approaches, her adrenaline rises. It halts her labor so that she can fight or take flight.[7]

And that, finally, explained to me why those Amish primips in the hospital had stalled labors. Frightened by an alien environment, their bodies seized up—making ready to flee. Surrounded by routines—all of which require compliance—they could not let go of neocortical considerations. Laboring in a brightly lighted, noisy, and intrusive setting, their bodies could not find their own rhythms. Feeling untrusted—"Hasn't she delivered yet?"—they turned against their bodies, questioning their performance. Pressured by me—"Do you feel like pushing?"—they began to will birth rather than to let it be.

The Inner Nature of Birth

Because of Odent's personal warmth and charm, one can forget the scientific detachment that characterized his work at Pithiviers. Odent's was basic research.[1] Instead of assuming that birth usually goes awry, Odent theorized that it might work. To test the possibility, he invented a kind of laboratory for observing birth in a state of nature. He stripped away customary interventions and eventually was able—as much as is possible in a human study—to see the original process. Observing it, applying available physiological information, he redescribed the birth process.

It seems to me that he designed the emotional environment at Pithiviers in a similar way. Instead of focusing on hospital needs, he turned to the woman the institution was serving. For the ordinary pregnant woman, he asked himself, what are pregnancy and birth about? His answer, as evidenced by those weekly gatherings, was that it is a family and community event. When he told that friend of mine that she should do what gave her pleasure during her pregnancy, he was confirming what she knew but was nervous about believing, that childbearing was in the normal, healthy order of things.

Odent's discoveries resulted from the principle that one should gather information from the source—in this case, women's births. In other words, Odent listened.

For me, there was only one lapse in Odent's account of birth. He did not not attempt to describe its intimate interior, the subtle moves of the muscle and bone. At first, the omission bothered me; I felt he might not be giving the woman enough care. The more I thought about it, however, the more I respected his restraint. In the first place, the midwives at Pithiviers probably did most of the basic care. In the second, he needed to find out how birth would behave if left to run its own course. Finally, and most significant, he implies that he stayed back because he was male. "Presently I am seriously considering leaving obstetrics," he writes in *Birth Reborn.* "This is at a time when male obstetricians would do well to retire progressively and restore childbirth to women."[2]

Because I have not felt restrained in the same way as Odent, however, I have had daily, intimate contact with birthing bodies. Employing Odent's principle of taking my information from women, I add where he demurred.

As a practitioner, I am guided by the strengths in my material. Like a cabinetmaker eyeing the pattern in wood, like a seamstress feeling the weight of a fabric, I search for the design of birth implicit in a woman. I can anticipate a birth best when I concentrate on information that comes to me through my hands. I glide them up over the bathed and talced mound of a woman's belly. In first-time mothers, when I pull my hands down, tracing the path the baby will take, I feel smooth, strong muscles and a baby who rides in a taut pouch. With experienced birthers, I can close my eyes and feel the revelation of work done, of skin that has stretched and reknit, of muscles that have spread and drawn back together. I can feel tenacious parts and those that are more lax. I can anticipate muscular dynamics. I can feel whether there is a good pool of waters, whether the baby has sufficient mass, and how vital it is.

I probe for the baby's head or bottom riding above a pubic bone. Placing my right hand on the hard, softballlike mass there and putting my left on the corresponding ball just below a rib cage, I ask a woman to take a deep breath. As her abdominal muscles relax, I can rock what is, most often, the baby's head. If it is not a little free, this mass, I'd suspect it might be the baby's bottom I am trying to wag and so reverse my maneuver. Later in pregnancy, I look for the head or bottom to slip deeper into the pelvic purse and get stodgy. When it's dropped out of reach, I can pretty much exclude placenta praevia, which means hemorrhage, and cord prolapse, which means the cord gets squeezed off during birth.

I try to pay attention to a woman's responses during these examinations, to the way she turns her head when I touch her, for example. I listen for small comments she might make—a passing remark about a pain here or a mention of something in her family's birth history. I watch her partner to find out how he responds to the examination. Thus I can keep what I teach in line with what a couple needs to know. I place a doptone on a woman's belly so we can hear the reassuring whoosh of the baby's heartbeat, the rush of placental blood, and the gurgling of the amniotic sea.

The body at birth is not static, but expressive and malleable. From the way a woman holds herself, I read how her body is responding to labor. If her eyes are wide and frantic, if her jaw is jammed down into her shoulders, her mouth pulled tight, her voice strained, her shoulders clamped in over her chest, her hands gripping one another, and her knees clenched, then we have to warm her up, teach her some techniques for being comfortable with her body while it is in labor. Like soaking wood in water, a long, warm bath can loosen her joints and transform them to a more elastic state. Her head drops back, floating freely, her hands dangle, her knees fall open. Her mouth softens and lets out throaty sounds, her breathing deepens and lengthens and the ease ripples down, as if warm and oiled, releasing the tension in her pelvis and cervix. I smooth my hands down her back in long slow sweeps, like stroking a cat, and my hand motions seem to carry over to her muscles, which begin to glide, sinuous, riding with the contractions as one rides a canoe over deep, slow waters. She begins to labor with the current of her body.

The body is malleable and birth is dynamic. Contractions, like hands kneading, close on the baby, whose moving mass then pressures the pelvis, causing it to spread; presses on the cervix, which gives way. We have three forces, which interplay: the power of contractions, the baby's body, and the expandable passage. None of these can be considered separately; they form and re-form in relationship to each other; they touch, respond, intertwine, converse, accommodate, embrace. It may be most appropriate to think of the process as dance.

The pelvis seems to be hard, set, stiff, measurable, unforgiving as an iron pot, but in fact it is flexible; it is webbed with leathery joints and can move. Sometimes I see swelling in the small of the back and know that the baby's head is ramming against a bony ledge. I ask the woman to squat down and to grip her husband's hands or the end of the bed for balance. I drop down in back of her, slip my fingers around the wingtips of her pelvis, place my knee in the small of her back and press. The pelvis, like a bow, springs the baby's head off the shelf and lets it slide down onto the lower curve of backbone that will guide it out.

The Spirit in Birth

Birth is infinitely dynamic. We cannot adequately understand it by naming anatomical parts and describing physiological processes, nor are we done when we describe its choreography. Birth functions in the context of mind and spirit. They act directly on birth and give it the complexity we associate with life. When we acknowledge this, we invite the power of birth.

Becca, John's wife, weighed ninety-five pounds and was as shy as a blade of new grass. Her skin was translucent; her bones were slender and fine as light. Fragility dominated her being, easily overwhelming the mere, plain fact that her pregnancy was normal. I could not imagine her having the capacity to throw her baby out. I could not think how to embolden her. The only way I could comfort myself was to dwell on her hot-ember hair and all the passion that superstition credits to redheaded women, but even that didn't really do, because she wore it as all Amish women do, carved in a center part and pulled back into a humble, restricted, "It's only me" knot.

Her husband, John, whom I wanted as an ally, was of the rough-and-tumble, dog tail–pulling type. I wished he would evoke some pacing lioness in her, but all he could do was poke her in the ribs. At childbirth classes, she blushed and he feigned indifference.

When the call came, I went out and found her coiled on her couch. When she pulled her skirt up and I saw a cupped-out space underneath her navel, I knew we had our share of work ahead. The baby was in what we call a "persistent posterior position," which means that labor may be long and back pain relentless. If our little Becca continued to conceal herself, as she seemed bound to do, the baby would stay in retreat and her energy would pour out, wasted. If she continued to curl up like a snail in its shell, we would be undone. Her eyes, I noticed, wandered over to John, beseeching his attention.

"You know," I said to her experimentally, "when you're canning pears, you sometimes shake the jar to get the halves to find their space?"

She nodded.

"Well, that's what we need to do for your baby. Jiggle him up a little, so his head can find the easy way out."

"How should I do that, Penny?" she asked, without a trace of confidence.

And John sat, careless as the devil, in a lounge chair by the window.

As I looked over at him, thinking about giving one of his casually flung out legs a good kick, I noticed the window behind him. It framed sunlight and a pasture that spilled down to a spot in a stream where the water coiled and made a pool. Ducks glided about on it. Feeling drawn to it myself, I said I thought it might be well for Becca to take a walk, on the condition that John go along. "You'll have to hold her hand so she doesn't fall, of course, and let her lean up against you when she has a contraction."

"We often walk down by the creek," he said, agreeably and comfortably—as if this was something he knew how to do. And so I left them alone for a while.

When I returned some time later, Becca was serving sandwiches. She raised hers to her mouth, apparently determined—per my instructions—to keep up her strength. Try as she might, she could not comply, and when I said she needn't eat if she didn't want to, she dropped her sandwich on her plate and her head on her arms. I looked hopefully at John, thinking that he might, by now, be following her reactions, but instead he was picking up her sandwich. As soon as he finished it, however, he rose with purpose, went into the bathroom, and returned with a hairbrush. Standing behind Becca, he loosened the knot of her bandana, undid her hair, and let it unfurl in red licks around her shoulders. Then he ran his fingertips gently up the side of her head, gathered a mass of her hair in one hand and sank the brush deep into its thick waves with the other. As he brushed, her head swayed gently. Her neck became loose and languid, and the sighs that flushed out of her were heavy.

Seeing that they were finding their way, I slipped as quickly as I could out into the yard and down to the stream, where I sat and waited for an outcome utterly beyond my control. When the sun dropped out of sight and I saw the flash and glow of a lantern lighting in the kitchen window, I rose, thinking that I had better go back in to work. Even as I gathered myself up, however, I stopped: Music was coming from the house. Music, so alien in an Amish household, coming out of this one, streaming out of windows, lapping down over the pasture, trailing into the stream. I stood a long time—unthinkable to break the thread of melody—then found that it was strong and continuous and so I followed it to its source. On my toes, peering in the farmhouse window, I saw Becca, head high and proud, red hair streaming and gallant down her back. She was pacing round the kitchen table, John following her, now playing "Swing Low, Sweet Chariot" on his harmonica.

I turned away once more and leaned against the clapboards while more songs followed and until the music drained away; until I heard Becca's groan. As I went in, John was helping her to bed; then he held her hand, smoothed her forehead, and ultimately he cradled her shoulders in his arms. In that position she threw out a boy baby, whom John reached for, held, and gave over to her.

Discouraging Birth

Becca's john, Michel Odent, and I made one discovery in common: that it is in the nature of birth to benefit from respect. John became so sensitive to his wife that he heard the rhythms of her body and transposed them into music. Michel Odent so respected the genius of the process that he stood back, concerned about tainting it. I took an approach more like John's in trying to learn the language of a particular woman's birth in order to accompany her through it.

Wherever we encounter caregivers who defer to birth, we find startlingly good outcomes. Midwives at the Frontier Nursing Service have managed nineteen thousand births for women from the back hills of Tennessee. Since 1955, they haven't had a maternal death, and since 1971 their perinatal mortality rate has averaged six per thousand, or less than half the average of the rest of the country.[1]

Since 1973, Dr. Mayer Eisenstein and his associates at Homefirst Medical Practice in Chicago have attended nearly 9,000 births.

Eighty-seven of these births have been at home and the remainder in the hospital. Of the clients who came to the practice during their pregnancies, the cesarean section rate was 4 percent. The practice's episiotomy rate was 1.2 percent and the perinatal mortality rate 3.3 per thousand.[2]

Dr. John Stevenson, an Australian doctor who discovered birth working in women's homes, has managed 1,190 births. Again, no maternal deaths, a perinatal mortality rate of 12.6 per thousand (against an Australian national average of 14.7 per thousand), and a transfer rate of 4.9 percent.[3]

The Home Birth Service of Los Angeles reports on 857 clients, of whom 92.6 percent delivered at home. They've had no maternal or perinatal deaths and 2.6 percent of their clients had cesarean sections.[4]

Probably the best-disciplined study to date is reported in a 1989 article in *The New England Journal of Medicine.* It is based on statistics gathered on 11,814 women who were admitted to birth centers for labor and delivery care. Of these women, 15.8 percent were transferred to hospital care during or soon after labor and birth and 4.4 percent of the transferred women had cesareans. The intrapartum (after labor has begun) and neonatal death rate (between birth and 28 days) for the babies of the 11,814 women was 1.3 per thousand.[5]

What these practitioners have in common is a belief in the efficacy of birth. In most cases, they need only use stethoscope, gloves, some gauze, all their senses, and two hands to see a baby out. They do not manage birth so much as they nourish it. They feed it. Being organic, it becomes more vital.

Making Failure

If birth succeeds when its innate character is respected, then the converse should be true: It should be more likely to fail when those who accompany a woman through pregnancy and birth fail to acknowledge what she and her body are expressing.

For an example of how birth can be undercut in this way, we return to Leslie, the woman whose birth we described in the first chapter. As she told the story, her birth began with the abortion she had as a young woman. It was a significant factor because it made her fear for her life and caused her to distrust her reproductive body.

If we look at the paralysis clinically, we can explain it two ways: The most likely is that the physician who conducted the abortion was incompetent in administering the anesthesia; the most remote is that Leslie suffered from an exotic reaction to hormonal change in her body. Since she had no other indications of irregular hormonal tendencies, however, and since the abortionist was both rude and cruel—not only did he yell at Leslie when she called to ask him questions but he refused to answer them—it seems reasonable to postulate that he made the mistake. Leslie, not having the expertise to analyze the experience clinically, drew a tentative conclusion: Her body betrayed her during a reproductive act.

Either because she instinctively trusted her body or because she was in the habit of assuming responsibility for her health, Leslie sought further for an explanation of the paralytic episode. When she asked her obstetrician, he gave her that neither-here-nor-there response: "I won't promise you something like that won't happen, but I don't think it will." His response wasn't wrong—he couldn't have been sure that poor anesthesia was the culprit—but it was insufficient. The obstetrician did not advocate for Leslie's body or her general good health, even though both would have been clinically appropriate.

Thus, the possibility of a womb-induced paralysis—and its association with death—lurked in Leslie's mind from early in pregnancy. From the beginning, birth was an uncertain ally: It might give her a much-wanted baby, but it was also a possible enemy, a carrier of death. Aware of her fear, perhaps wondering if it would forestall birth, thinking how to cope with it, Leslie gave herself the option of "taking something."

Given the facts she had to work with, Leslie made a responsible decision. She acknowledged her fear, she did not want to complicate her child's birth, and she decided she would dose herself if she had to. Unfortunately, the facts she had were distorted.

They were also incomplete. Leslie mentioned that her decision to take something was in line with her feminism. She said she saw no need for a woman to suffer just because she was performing a female function. She argued, quite correctly, that feminists had led the campaign for painkillers during birth for over a century.

What she missed, however, was that drugs that dull labor pain also diminish power and flatten energy. The *Physicians' Desk Reference* tells us that a hazard of Demerol, for example, is "respiratory depression and, to a lesser degree, circulatory depression." Furthermore, it advises that Demerol crosses from the mother's blood to the baby's and "causes depression of respiration and psychophysiologic functions in the newborn."

This is not new information. Birth practitioners for over a century have been concerned with the depressive effects of painkilling drugs in childbirth. For some reason, however, the information did not get to Leslie. At least she did not mention them.

Leslie began her labor in fear. Fear, we remember from Odent, inhibits labor. In spite of it, however, she willed herself through her early pains. She attached her head to her husband's shoulder and took strength from him and he, the only nonprofessional in attendance, gave her what is most needed during birth—acceptance and comfort. He nourished her.

The nurse, by contrast, did not suggest positions that might have made Leslie more comfortable, she did not apply the butt of her hand against Leslie's tailbone, which helps with back labor, she did not offer a shower or bath, which are known to diminish pain. Most glaringly, she (apparently) did not explain that the bolt of nausea Leslie felt (which stimulated her fear and her decision to take drugs) was an excellent sign. Far from indicating the onset of paralysis, the nausea indicated that Leslie's body was in vigorous labor.

Throughout her pregnancy and labor Leslie's body was underappreciated; similarly, her personal maturity and strength were not valued. The birth reflex itself was neglected. Indeed, the nurse happily offered to drug it. The doctor too. It is not too much to say that Leslie, at the most emotionally and physically vulnerable point in her labor, was guided into intervention.

And so she fell into that sludgy sleep, and when her husband woke her and asked her to breathe, she said, "Why should I?" The baby's heartbeat dropped because of the drugs in her system and because of the position of the cord. She couldn't put her strength into pushing her baby past her tailbone because she was only half alive. The doctor resorted to an episiotomy that required forty minutes to stitch, and to forceps, which neither Leslie nor her husband had wanted.

Women Explain Failure

Most women do not criticize their birthcare directly. They'll make a tangential comment, as Leslie did with her remark about being forgotten, or lump the whole event in the category of "necessary trial" and forget it. Others maintain that the way one gives birth is a trifling matter anyway; what counts is the lifetime of parenting. A minority, however, can't deny, accept, or forget. The feeling of having been assaulted opens wide wounds in them.

The Cesarean Prevention Movement (CPM) is an education/support organization for such women.[6] CPM sponsors conferences, provides literature, patches networks together, and responds to individual women all over the country who are interested in preventing or avoiding cesarean section or who are healing from it. In 1987, over five thousand women contacted CPM offices.

Because the organization actively invites women to express their feelings about birth, their conference in August 1987 provided us with an opportunity to hear what most women don't talk about. Certainly, the program—designed to provide information and to help parents heal—encouraged such openness.

About two hundred young parents, babies in their arms or toddling by their side, assembled in the lecture hall the first morning. Blankets were tossed onto the carpeted floor; infants were deposited, murmuring and drooling, upon them. An occasional toddler would crawl up the aisle, up the steps to the base of the podium, turn, and sit facing us, in oblivious command. Conference participants had agreed that babies had some right of way. They also established that many of their number had traveled from several states away to attend the weekend conference. Most said that they felt profoundly wounded, victimized, and/or abused by the experience of cesarean section and that they wanted to heal.

Esther Zorn, president of CPM, reminded us before we began that there was no right and wrong to feel about a birth experience; that our discussion might be very painful for some; that we needed to accept one another; that we needed to relearn trust; and that our pain could help us. After some relaxation exercises, a facilitator asked the audience to respond to the question: "Why did this happen to me?"

"We let it happen because we are afraid to speak up."

"Women are afraid to say no to authority figures."

"We perceive ourselves as victims. We feel paralyzed."

"We feel we can't do anything, so we don't do anything [i.e., protect ourselves, ask questions or give birth]."

"We're afraid of our insides."

They felt they had been called upon to challenge, to defy, and to say no, and that they had failed. Their comments implied that they regretted not having prepared themselves to campaign for vaginal birth. They suggested that they thought they should have been able to labor, birth, and fight at the same time; that one should not just be strong, but *stronger* than the system that surrounded them.

The self-accusatory strain of their remarks helps explain why women might not be speaking out about their births. If women perceive cesarean as being a result of a character fault within themselves—"We were weak"—then they would be less likely to make a commotion about it. But setting that issue aside for the time being, and translating the question "Who's at fault?" to "What's at fault?" we find a remarkable congruence between their feelings about what would have made their births work and Odent's theories. The obstacle to birth, they were saying, was that they were not heard.

Suppose, then, that they could be heard. Suppose that they were not "afraid of their insides" or of "authority figures," what might they have expressed about birth? The facilitator asked, "What is birthing energy?"

"Tension."

"Love."

"Excitement."

"Camaraderie."

"Sacredness."

"Absorption."

"Power."

"Humility."

"Warmth."

"Beauty."

"Serenity."

"Birthing energy is self-birth."

"It is loving ourselves and our bodies."

"It connects each woman with all women, linking them through space and time."

"It is a feeling of the power of life let through."

Women described being swept up by a force larger than themselves. A river, birth was, always there, going on, unmindful of women and women unmindful of it, until its waters flushed in about their ankles. During labor, they stepped in. Its currents carried them to the other side. Birth was more powerful than a woman was. That was its meaning. Like surrendering to forests or mountain peaks of hosts of stars, an experience of communion. Too vast for words, igniting spirit.

How the women came up with the language they did is baffling. No one seemed to be coaching them, this audience of so many people who had experienced surgical, not natural birth, and yet they knew about the power of birth and that they had been prevented from experiencing it. It was an emotional morning.

In the afternoon, we turned to practical matters. At a panel presentation, "Reversing Cesarean Trends," we listened to Dr. Norbert Gleicher, chairman of the Mount Sinai Hospital Medical Center in Chicago. The 25 percent cesarean rate in the United States was unacceptable, Gleicher said. We should be seeing numbers like 6 to 10 percent. To get them, he and members of his department were requiring women who had had previous cesareans to attempt to labor and give birth vaginally. (That women attempt VBAC, or vaginal birth[7] after cesarean section, was not a universal requirement. There are instances where vaginal birth is not an option.) They were also requiring a second opinion on all decisions to perform cesarean. Using these methods, Mt. Sinai had reduced its cesarean rate from 16 percent to 13 percent in one year.[8]

Gleicher urged the audience to assume some of the responsibility for bringing about change and, in that spirit, suggested they concentrate on educating doctors rather than attacking them. They would do well to remember that physicians had not gotten into the habit of doing cesareans because they were vicious people, but because they believed that cesareans were in the best interests of their patients. While this might not be clinically correct, generally speaking, it did not make the doctors bad. It just made them wrong.

Remedying the mistake, he advised, would require time and patience. "In science, it takes a while to discover your errors." Furthermore, the American College of Obstetricians and Gynecologists was "conservative by nature." The best way to move the doctors along, he advised, was by presenting them with "hard facts," some of which he provided.

Dr. Gleicher's message might have been better received had he underplayed some of the other factors that he felt contributed to the high rates of cesarean section. The members of this audience, many of whom were still feeling raw, couldn't be expected to muster much sympathy when he told them how "very unpleasant" it was for a physician to face a deposition; or how the doctor, his head on the block of a legal guillotine, may practice "defensive," i.e., surgical medicine. They didn't respond well when he mentioned that "American midwifery may have caused some of the problems . . . by creating a certain antagonism between doctors and patients." Nor when he observed that women themselves could be driving up the section rate by "demanding surgical solutions." While many of these were legitimate points, they didn't sit well with this particular audience.

Maybe, too, there was something subtly affronting about Dr. Gleicher's presentation. Something obstructive about body language, something authoritarian in his tone. But given his deeds—here was an obstetrician who had taken decisive steps to reduce cesarean section, a doctor who had leaped where science crawled, a liberal where the American College was conservative—the response of the audience was peculiar.

As he talked, people muttered. A few blurted out challenges. We heard a repressed hiss behind us. When the audience was asked for questions, they hurled accusations back. The woman next to us turned her shoulder to Dr. Gleicher and, unsolicited, gave us a short, vitriolic speech about the male-dominated, female-dominating arrogance of the medical profession.

Hard as we tried to remain objective, we knew we were emotionally aligned with the crowd. The only difference between us and them (we thought) was that intellectually we respected Dr. Gleicher's achievements and thought he ought to have been applauded for them, which he wasn't.

We worked this peculiar event over for some months following the convention. Were we offended because we'd spent the morning talking about birth as a transcendent event and that Dr. Gleicher had been given the task of speaking about its merely medical aspects? Having soared, had we resented being reminded that our flight was also a matter of wing shapes, metal selection, and angles of ascent. Would we have been less discontent if Dr. Gleicher had acknowledged the sublime? Or did our reaction have something to do with the way Dr. Gleicher held his head.

Then we ran across an article in *Parents* magazine called "Do Cesareans Save Lives?" Quoted in it, Dr. Gleicher was rebutting the opinion of certain doctors who said that the high cesarean rate was not entirely their doing; there were, for example, women who didn't want to try a vaginal birth after cesarean section. It was a point Gleicher himself had made.

While the other doctors in the article said you couldn't go against women's wishes, Gleicher disagreed: "I have a philosophical problem with that," he said. "We can't let patients dictate incorrect medical procedure."[9]

This gets us into a subtle problem. The doctor does have responsibility for the medical conduct of a labor and birth, and the patient does not have knowledge equal to that of the physician. But, as we will see later, women who feel that their caregivers have responded to their concerns are generally grateful to rely on their judgment. The conflict seems to arise when the woman feels she is being silenced.

Which goes a long way in explaining why the women reacted as they did. In those first sessions, trying to understand why they'd ended up with surgery, obviously speaking from their hearts, the women said they had had cesareans because they couldn't or didn't make themselves heard. If they had been heard, they would have had access to the "power of life let through."

In his presentation, Dr. Gleicher may not have illustrated his ability to listen. Admirable as his achievements were, consistent as they were with the organization's goals, he may have conveyed an impression that doctors could and should—to use his verb—"dictate" birth decisions.

If this is his stance, he is not alone. In October of 1988, the Associated Press released the following story: "Breaking with a seventy-year old tradition, the American College of Obstetricians and Gynecologists declared yesterday that women who have had a baby by Caesarean section generally should deliver subsequent children by normal birth."

"[S]hould," it says. Not "women should be able to" or "women should be helped to" but women "should." It is possible that the word should was being used in the predictive sense—women probably will, but when one reflects on birth stories like Leslie's and Mary's, when one considers how brave CPM members thought they had to be to express their thoughts, one suspects a prescriptive meaning. In the climate of birth today, the word *should* sounds like an order, one that turns a deaf ear to messages coming from the source.[10]

The Failure of the Solution

The problem of the successful birth might appear to be solved. We've said that if a caretaker imposes too much upon a woman, disregarding information he or she might take from her, then the power of birth diminishes. If a caretaker listens to a woman, demonstrates confidence in the birth process, turns the lights down, is kind, patient, and skilled, then power invades and the woman gives birth naturally and satisfactorily.

Unfortunately, it isn't that simple. Even when given most of these advantages, women do end up with medicalized births, and the midwives who assist them are the first to say so. To get at the reasons, we invited six midwives, representing forty-six years of experience, to talk with us. Taken together, the women had covered the continent: San Francisco General to North Central Bronx, rural Mississippi to urban Chicago. One of the midwives had trained in England, two currently were running their own birth center, several had worked among the poor, and one, Sue Yates, had just completed her term as President of the American College of Nurse-Midwives (ACNM).

For all their time in institutions, they still spoke of women as moms and not as "prolapsed cords"; they referred to babies rather than "neonates." They believed birth could be a wonderful experience and a couple of them referred to it as an act of God. They felt it could empower women. They said "something does happen" when a woman gives birth, something out of the ordinary, even transcendent. And they spoke bitterly and vehemently of practitioners, whether midwives or obstetricians, who "virtually raped" women or "gorped babies."

They were convinced that the women who came to them had a better chance at a good birth. Ruth Shiers summed it up with a story about a client, a PhD psychologist who took her baby to the Y for swimming classes with other young mothers. Inevitably they compared birth stories. The psychologist reported back to Ruth that she was "the only one in the room who felt positive about my birth experience."

When we asked them what they did to help birth work, their answers circled the same orb as Odent's, Penny's, and those of the women at the CPM Conference. Katie Head, a stocky, dark-haired woman with a penchant for roving the room and shoving her hands in the front pockets of her pants, said, "I think I give the woman energy."

Her birth center partner Ruth added, "I'm exhausted after a long labor."

The English midwife M. J. Hanafin tossed in, "It is energy that you give out and she gives back so that the two intermingle."

"I can't stand to talk about birthing energy," Sue Yates, the former ACNM executive said, somewhat tartly. "The hippie stuff. The opening of the flower. Humph. But I can remember a lot of time going into a labor that I would put a hand on a shoulder, a hand on a hip, and something happens. I don't know what it is . . . but I do know there is something in the hands."

Pat Payne, an outrageous Texan who remembered looking down between her legs when her daughter was about to be born and hearing the doctor say, "Do you want me to deaden IT?" said, "You give everything you've got. You pick her up, you love her, you embrace her, you cheer her on, you scold her, you seduce her, you do everything you can do to get the woman to do for herself."

"She lets go and trusts in her labor."

"She becomes well directed toward her goal."

"If I was a hippie," someone said, throwing a glance at Sue, "I'd say you hold the light for them."

When you support women as you describe, we asked, does it ensure that they will give birth naturally? Sylphlike blond Connie Sinclair had just arrived. "Putting aside all those women who . . . can get through with love and encouragement and all that, there is the other group that want anesthesia, who do not want that labor," she said, grabbing at a coil of hair that had slipped over her shoulder and flipping it back. "We had a patient who came in around thirty-four weeks with a breech. We gave her exercises [to encourage the baby to turn to the head-down position] but she didn't do them . . . and she wasn't telling us that she wasn't doing them. . . . She ended up with a c-section for breech. Afterward, she said to us, 'I had no intention of going through labor.' "

M. J. noted: "My sister has a very low pain threshold. She has two sisters who are midwives. She told us she knew she was supposed to have her baby naturally and all that, but she chose a cesarean and she's happy. No regrets. It hasn't made any difference in her mothering."

Katie said, "We've had a couple of people who've had perfectly horrible labors. Posterior, on and on and on and they said, 'I want to go to the hospital [and have drugs] because I can't endure it.' "

"Pain interferes with some mothers' relationship with their child," Sue observed. "They hate that child for giving them pain. An epidural may help a relationship. A cesarean may result."

M. J. said, "I saw it [epidurals] work in San Francisco. If you can time it just right so she feels to push, she gets mad when the pain comes, she pushes the kid right out, and you get a healthy kid and a happy mother. And she's empowered."

Pat added, "The wonderful thing about where we are in history today is that we've got the choices. The question is whether we use them wisely."

Connie: "The dignity of the midwifery birth is that it allows women to make the choices for themselves. That's empowering women for their own circumstances."

"The essence of midwifery is flexibility," M. J. said.

What seemed notable to us about the midwives' remarks was the priority they placed on women having the choice. Their allegiance to her and her needs was impeccable. In application, however, their adherence to the support-the-woman's choice philosophy raised two problems: One was clinical, the other fundamental to our interest in finding out why most American women cannot give birth as Amish women do.

The clinical conundrum goes as follows. If it is true that women have more difficulty giving birth if their wishes are not respected, then it is clinically sound to honor their requests. On the other hand, honoring a request for pain medication is tantamount to providing support for a process that starts innocently enough with an epidural but which can lead to cesarean.

It's often called the cascade of interventions and we saw it at work in Leslie's birth. The painkilling drug slowed down her system and compromised her capacity to push the baby out. In other hands, or in another ten minutes, Leslie might well have ended up with a cesarean. Cesarean has hazards for the mother: "Maternal morbidity (disease) rates are generally five to ten times higher after cesarean delivery than after vaginal delivery."[11] Cesarean has disadvantages for the baby: "There is a higher mortality . . . for infants delivered by a cesarean and far more respiratory complications."[12] Although the reasons behind these statistics are just beginning to be understood, studies are showing that the process of moving through the birth canal squeezes fluid from the baby's lungs. Furthermore, the stresses of vaginal birth "help a baby's lungs mature, regulate body temperature and send blood to the brain and heart."[13]

Although she knows the benefits of the vaginal birth and the disadvantages of the cesarean, a midwife still cannot impose natural birth upon a woman. It is impossible. So the midwife follows the only course left to her: She gives a woman complete information, offers abundant reassurance, and then supports a woman's decisions. The realities of birth, not moral considerations, put the responsibility for the decisions on the woman.

That woman, as we have seen, has her own realities. "You can't divorce birth from conditioning. . . . It's a very strong, very unusual, very motivated woman who deviates from [the traditional hospital, medicated] birth," Kate explained. "A woman is not a blank page," Sue Yates added.

Which leads us to the pivotal problem. Why do women have so little confidence in their capacity to give birth naturally? Or, to put it another way, why don't they *want* to try?

PART II

LEGACIES

Introduction

Listening to the women at the CPM Conference, one might
make a quick judgment about the reasons why women lack confidence in their birthing bodies. Their comments on their perceived
failures have such a familiar ring—"We failed because we didn't
believe in ourselves" or, to put the blame elsewhere, "We failed
because male medical professionals didn't respect us." We might say
then that women's lack of confidence about their birthing capacities,
their dependence today on physicians and technology, is just another
tiresome example of how women in our culture have been disre-
spected and diminished and how women have internalized these
destructive attitudes.

If we did say that, we would be partly right. As we will see, our
culture's estimate of what women are capable of has influenced
women's beliefs about their bodies and their behavior at birth. But
it would be deceiving to quit there. Women have acted aggressively

and energetically in shaping birth history. Not only did they have major responsibility for the conduct of birth in the last century, but they have actively participated in the decisions that have led to changes in birth management since then. They have chosen, just as women today choose, how to give birth and always with good reasons. Their decisions arose less from a poor sense of self and more from the hard realities of birth.

Remembering:
"The Great Emergency"

WOMEN USED to die in childbirth. Before doctors became so well trained, before hospitals, before modern medicine, they died in shocking numbers. In the nineteenth century, women missed their period, they felt nauseous, their breasts grew tender, and they wondered if the next nine months would be their last. One spent one's pregnancy "preparing the layette for the newcomer by reusing the layette of those who, dead or alive, had come before, and, more discreetly, collecting each time in one of her dresser drawers bits and pieces of her own deathbed attire on which were pinned last wishes in case God would, on this occasion, call her to Him."[1]

Babies got stuck in their mothers' pelves, which might have been distorted by inadequate diets. Rachitic pelvis, it's called, and in the old days the only way to save the mother's life was to dismember the infant in utero and remove it in pieces. Mothers died from complications of tuberculosis which, in the nineteenth century, was epidemic.

Poor urban women died because their bodies were compromised by unclean water and milk, poor diet, and overwork. Rich women faltered because they subsisted on fashionable proteinless diets and because they wore corsets that grievously distorted their reproductive anatomy. All classes of women died from the postpartum infection called childbed fever.

Women regularly attended friends and neighbors who suffered horribly and died. Birth in nineteenth-century America was as it has been from time immemorial: a woman's concern. "In most cultures," write anthropologist Margaret Mead and psychologist Niles Newton, "daughters, sisters, mothers, mothers-in-law, co-wives and other relatives and friends are regarded as the natural helpers of a woman during the childbearing process. Assistance before and after the baby is born is almost always in the hands of other women."[2]

It was no different in America. "Dearest mother mine," wrote one pregnant woman in 1890, "all would be complete if you were here." Her mother responded, "Dearie, I wish I were there to thoroughly rub olive oil upon you [sic] hips, your groin muscles, your abdominal muscles all through—in short all the muscles that are to be called upon to yield, and be elastic at the proper time. See how reasonable it seems that they should be helped to yield, to do their work if they are kneaded by the strong hand of a mother, while olive oil is being *freely applied.*"[3]

Women used to travel hundreds of miles to be with their mothers when the time came. If they couldn't get to her, they turned to other women. "Women would write and speak to each other intimate details of confinement related care; they would confide their innermost thoughts about their coming motherhood." When the hour of crisis arrived, women expected to be taken care of by other women, whether they claimed to be midwives or not. In frontier settings, the male's duty was to round up the neighboring women, who were deeply obligated to respond. "Women went to considerable sacrifice to help their birthing relatives and friends, they interrupted their lives."[4]

When women arrived in one another's homes, their skirts and petticoats whisking, they crowded the men to parlor corners. Carrying their overnight satchels, bearing herbs and oils, tying on their authoritative aprons, and brimming with opinions, the women bustled, they slid pots on the stove, they disciplined children, they rummaged for rags and sheets, they plumped pillows, they negotiated strategies, and they commanded quiet. Having lives to bring forth and sisters to save, they determined what the distant, pacing men should and shouldn't be told.

It was mid-nineteenth century when doctors began to enter the birthplace. Women, midwives in their number, did not exactly welcome the new-minted experts. The birthplace was their territory, after all, and as tightly held as a traditional holiday kitchen. Furthermore, doctors had little to recommend them. Frequently they were men who'd taken a few weeks off from forge or farm to attend an unaccredited school where they read textbooks and listened to lectures from others who were hardly better educated than they. During their training, it was morally unthinkable for them to witness a birth.

Women, by contrast, had been learning since childhood how to care for the sick, the laboring, and the dying. They knew a lot in comparison to the doctors, including their limits. When they heard rumors of instruments that could be used to pull a baby out and the riveting news of the painkilling effects of chloroform and ether, they were interested.

One thinks sympathetically of the male doctors who first ventured into the steamy coven of women. Alone, poorly trained, and of mediocre social status, they would have been a pathetic sight. Standing in women's bedrooms, holding their little battered black bags in their hands, they must have seemed more like supplicants than priests. They entered on probation. After all, one husband wrote, the doctor's "life has not been in jeopardy. Except in sympathy his nerves have not been racked, his muscles strained, his joints wrenched, his fibers torn, his blood spilled."[5]

Indeed, the early doctors must have trembled as women did when women first broke the barricades protecting the corporate boardroom: sweaty with fear of nonacceptance, worried about adequacy, and anxious about crossing gender lines. To succeed, they adopted the standing culture of the workplace. So one doctor described how he "sat up all night and talked *scandal* with some Cornish women in attendance."[6]

Quite literally fighting for lives, the doctors and the women negotiated information and decisions, the women bringing the authority of experience and doctors offering what they'd learned from books. Doctors tapped into sweat wisdom. They observed the natural course of birth, imbibed the old wives' tales, and grew in their understanding of the process. Many learned quickly to be distrustful of the broad use of ether and chloroform to ease pain. In their medical journals they wrote that anesthetics could "increase the danger of hemorrhage, could lead to protracted labor, could decrease uterine contractions, and could cause a newborn breathing difficulty."[7]

But no one completely rejected the drugs. One could not see a woman's excruciating, insoluble pain dispatched with ether or chloroform and ignore them. They used them, experimented with them, even though it meant rejecting the religious tradition that said that the agony of labor, the "pain and suffering beyond bearing," was a woman's penalty for being a daughter of Eve. When women, seeing the beneficence of the vapors, subsequently claimed the privilege of relief, they were not giving up power to men, they were refusing the ancient punishment for being born female.

They also took their chances with forceps. Yes, there were times when the instruments were disastrously applied: An unskilled or overly aggressive physician might grab a woman's flesh with the head of a baby and, in pulling, tear her catastrophically. But one could not watch a birth-resistant child safely taken by forceps and deny the miracle.

And doctors were learning: One physician wrote in a 1897 medical journal: "I see so many doctors who, in almost every case of obstetrics they get—put on forceps to 'hasten delivery and shorten the woman's suffering.' I am very positive that this frequent use of forceps is abuse."[8] Another, of a similar mind, recommended to his students that they "leave the forceps at home when they traveled to attend laboring women, so that if they were tempted to use them, they would have to travel back to their homes first, thus giving the parturient more time to achieve the delivery without them."[9] There were vigorous debates in the journals about the use of ether and chloroform.

But with all the experimentation, even with the combining of practical experience and new science, women died. At the turn of the century, one woman died for every 154 births. If a woman had five babies, which was common, her chance of surviving her reproductive life was one in thirty.[10] Doctors and midwives, mothers and neighbors, with equal frequency, watched the life ebb out of women and felt babies grow cold in their hands. All had to drop their heads: God giveth and God taketh away.

So when we wonder why women today have as little confidence as they do in the ability of their bodies to give birth naturally, we do well to remember that the last time women regularly gave birth at home, where lights were low, among people who were kind and with limited medical attention, their chances of survival were not good.

Miraculous Interventions

At the turn of the century, though, things began to look much more promising. Prodding the underside of the sad, familiar statistics were the beginnings of a medical revolution. Bits of medical knowledge had been tossed into the scientific sea until their number reached critical mass. Particular experimental findings collided, they cross-fertilized, and we were upended by explosive discovery. In the 1880s, in a rush of metal and glass, came the stethoscope, laryngoscope, opthalmoscope. In the same decade, the organisms responsible for tuberculosis, cholera, typhoid, and diphtheria were isolated. Not long after, we had the X ray, spirometer, electrocardiograph, as well as some chemical and bacteriological technologies.

Limited as their healing value was at the time, the inventions and discoveries advanced us. Naming and identifying are the beginning of a data base, which is the foundation for comparison and cross-comparison. One discovery is not only a prod for the next; each is an elixir for the hopeful imagination. The cascade of findings held out promise, reasons to believe, to risk. For the first time in history, humans dared think about reversing disease and defying death in a relatively reliable manner; they could think of wiping out the old familiar plagues, including that of childbirth.

We reevaluated ourselves and our responsibilities. If ordinary men, who were not the Son of God, could anticipate saying, "Take up your bed and walk," then it was incumbent upon them to proceed as rapidly as possible in that direction. This nation, never fearful of new frontiers, blessed with resources, mortgaged itself to medical advancement and put its faith in medical researchers and practitioners.

We were well positioned for this enterprise, which so thoroughly claimed our imaginations. As Paul Starr explains in *The Social Transformation of American Medicine*, [11] universities had been changing from centers for antique and elitist learning into pragmatic institutions, geared up to educate Americans for the increasingly complex requirements of daily life in the modern world. With an infusion of cash (fortuitously accumulated by corporations and waiting for philanthropic bestowal), upscaled universities were meant to release medicine from its crude past and thrust it into a healthier future. Out went the make-do medical school, those self-styled colleges of medicine that required only a couple of months of study for a couple of years in a row, where learning came from quasi-scientific books and was presented by practitioners, who (self-servingly) charged the students by the head. Out went all the sloppy licensing practices that allowed those colleges to continue and their students to practice.

They were replaced by great modern universities like Harvard and Johns Hopkins. At those institutions, medical students were expected to arrive with requisite undergraduate degrees. Once admitted, they stayed for several years, honing their skills. They attended lectures by salaried professionals, bent over microscopes in well-equipped laboratories, and practiced their craft on real humans under the critical eye of their seniors. Research institutes appended to the universities pumped intellectual adrenaline into their systems. The surge was at once sobering and heady.

Hospitals, which had existed primarily for those who didn't have a home and family care, were appropriated, thus providing students a place to practice their science and an opportunity to experiment. Patients of all kinds, including parturient women, were drawn in. At first it was the urban poor who were cared for in hospitals, but before long, middle-class women were attracted to them.

It was not a matter of submitting to men. The women were fighting the hazards of birth. If that meant facing a new and strange environment, it would have been a small price to pay. Why cling to the old ways: a sentimental and abstract notion of preserving women's tradition, women's turf? Why wait for one's mother to come, wait on, and attend them: mothers for whom urban, not rural homes, made no room? Why wait upon the neighbors, who were not compelled as their forebears had been, to give assistance? Why trust Nature, who had proved herself to be so callous? How could one bear to wonder if a modern doctor in a hospital, about whom one had read, might not have been able to save one's stillborn child?

Indeed, so promising were doctors' powers that lapses in performance were endured in good faith. The obstetrical wing of American medicine, in fact, had stumbled in the first thirty years of the century. Having drawn women into the hospital to give birth in the modern way, physicians were bewildered to discover that infant and maternal mortality rates did not decline. Science had uncommon trouble taming the streptococcus bacilli which, despite seemingly scrupulous sanitary measures, carried infection from sick patients to the birthing ones, as if magnetized by birth bruises and lacerations. For the first forty years of the twentieth century, urban (more hospitalized) women were much more likely to die in childbirth than their rural (more home-birthing) cousins.[12]

Complicating the matter, doctors tended to intervene too much and too soon in the birth process. Some were still administering drugs in unmeasured amounts and clamping forceps on babies heads before they had descended into the birth canal. Retrospectively, we can accuse them of hubris—of overestimating their ability to improve upon nature—but that neglects the deservedly poor reputation of nature at the time, not to mention the resurrective temptations inherent in the quest.

Then, too, there was a tragic historical coincidence, the mingling of hubris with certain sexist attitudes of the time. The middle-class women upon whom doctors experimented in those early days of hospital birth were perceived as being frailer than women had ever been thought to be. Their water-hauling, wood-chopping capacities had been, in popular opinion, bred out of them and, having become overcivilized, they were said to have lost their durability and resiliency.

Gallantly, physicians attempted to protect them from birth. Dr. Joseph DeLee, an obstetrician who devoted his life to improving the care of women during childbirth (taking considerable professional risk in the process) reflected this attitude. Writing in the first volume of the *American Journal of Obstetrics and Gynecology* in 1920, he observed that "only a small minority of women escape damage during labor." To protect them, he "recommended reducing birth to predictable patterns by using outlet forceps and episiotomy routinely and prophylactically in normal deliveries. DeLee sedated the parturient with scopolamine, allowed the cervix to dilate, gave ether during the second stage, performed an episiotomy, and lifted the fetus out with forceps. He then extracted the placenta, gave ergot to help the uterus contract, and stitched the perineal cut."[13] Not to say that DeLee was an insensitive practitioner; he was protective of women in his gentlemanly, Victorian way and prescribed certain teacakes for women to take during recovery. For all his efforts, women still died in discouraging numbers.

Mercilessly, the profession criticized itself for the problems they encountered with birth. "The New York Academy of Medicine, the Philadelphia County Medical Society, the White House Conference on Child Health and Protection, and countless individual practitioners went on record in the early 1930's proclaiming physicians themselves responsible for over half of America's preventable maternal deaths and claiming that hospitals exacerbated these dangers."[14] Identifying sloppy aseptic (sterile) techniques, wanton use of anesthetics, and "meddlesome" obstetrical practices as the problems, they set about correcting them. They established regulations to control the overuse and misuse of drugs, they established minimum delivery standards, and got a hold on asepsis. By the mid-forties they were able to announce that the hospital "was not associated with higher rates of puerperal [childbed] death."[15]

Thus obstetricians acquitted themselves with an honor worthy of confidence. Certainly they tangled with the side effects of their discoveries, obviously they failed, but, notably spirited, self-disciplined, and determined, they confronted their failures and mastered the painful obscurities. Never letting go of the promise of medical science, they isolated, investigated, and defeated many of its discoverable flaws. The effort was heroic, laudatory, and, as it is today, fully mesmerizing.

But for women carrying children in those decades, the message one could take from the offensive against birth was not reassuring. If physicians—propelled by high purpose and equipped with the best educations the world could offer—if they were undone by birth, then the process had to be frighteningly lethal.

Common Practice

In our medical quest, we pushed aside an important source of information. We deprived ourselves of accumulated knowledge about the relatively undisturbed birth. With a vengeance.

The case against midwives, the one group of people who could speak for the efficacies of natural birth, was overwhelming. In the heady days of scientific discovery, midwives, who were women and therefore judged incapable of thought, were said to be truculent, tradition-bound, and unscientific. Not only did they insist on sticking with the old, obviously faulty methods of delivering babies, but they played outright to superstition. As if flaunting objectivity, they honored local rituals and beliefs. They practiced as they had learned from their neighborhood mentors, they annointed babies as the local culture required, and wrapped them as illiterate grandmothers determined. Retrospectively, we might appreciate their service—we who are now sensitive to cultural issues, who say that birth has meaning in family tradition, and that caregivers serve well who serve the whole human. But in those days, the villain was raw death. Sociological niceties had not been invented and medical scientists could freely castigate midwives for their deference to arbitrary and foreign beliefs.

Midwives not only practiced unscientifically and thus weighed progress down, but by their willingness to serve poor women, they seemed to sabotage it. By giving home care to the less fortunate they deprived hospitals of the patients they needed to improve their techniques. If poor women stayed at home and had their babies with midwives, medical science could not acquire the necessary experience it needed. If scientists could not experiment, if student physicians could not practice their craft, we would remain stuck forever in the past. Did midwives, science might reasonably ask, not care for progress?

Economic factors, to be sure, invigorated some of those who challenged midwives. The physician who invested six to eight years on a medical education, equipped himself with every advanced technique, and charged accordingly, might well resent the midwife who learned to deliver babies from her great aunt (and charged accordingly). The very existence of such cheap care was an affront to the accomplishments of science and to the economic respectability that accrued to its practitioners. He sometimes resorted to less than honorable devices to make his complaint.

In what proportion these factors—sexist, classist, economic, and idealistic—mixed, is hard to say, but it's true that the campaign against midwives was marked by zealotry, ugliness, and, too often, gross insensitivity. Many immigrant midwives, for example, had been well trained in their home countries and were trusted by clients who appreciated cultural familiarities. Many of them were known to perform competently at the bedside—certainly as well as physicians, who were in the losing phase of the battle with the streptococcus bacilli—but these facts were ignored and immigrant midwives were uniformly vilified, called dirty, ignorant, drunk, etc. Ruthlessly, midwives' reputations were smeared by racist and elitist remarks. They were all like "granny" midwives, it was said, as if there was something revolting about the rural and often black women who learned their trade by necessity, who carried herbs and folk medicine into homes where doctors would not go.

It was not honorable. The campaign neglected the needs of poor women particularly; it was distorted by coarse prejudices and deranged by the raw ambition of the new science. What's worse, it wasn't necessary: As a nation we were committed to medical science and would have followed where it led us. It is regrettable, we can say now, that the practice of midwifery was slurred, because that has prevented us from understanding the strengths of the natural process, but the campaign was successful and midwives all but disappeared from public awareness between 1900 and 1930.

When they started to become visible again, midwives demonstrated what might be perceived as an uninstructable bent. Instead of imitating doctors, they continued in the old female tradition. Like the Sisters of Charity, like the founders of settlement houses, like visitors to the poor, like midwives before them, the new midwives took their practice to the poor, where they attended to seemingly paltry matters like nutrition and cleanliness as much as they attended birth.

Consider the history of the Maternity Center Association in New York City. Originally, its purpose was to distribute tuberculine-free milk to infants and toddlers of immigrants. In 1918, the association, keeping up with changes in thinking about public health, opened neighborhood prenatal clinics for the purpose of teaching women how to care for themselves and their infants—probably by offering information about diet and cleanliness. Astoundingly, the death rate for birthing women who attended the clinics dropped by 21.5 percent; the death rate for their babies dropped 29.2 percent.[16]

While this was clearly for the good, it was not the kind of news to capture middle-class imagination. There was no reason to think that what benefited the poor pregnant women of New York City would help women who, presumably, knew to wash and eat. The promise for middle- and upper-class women remained with physicians who wore "sanitary" white, prescribed medicines, had attractive offices, commanded hospitals, conducted dramatic surgeries, and swept away the pain of childbirth. The simple prenatal deeds of the good women at the Maternity Center Association could not compare; indeed, they might well have been considered irrelevant.

As unglamorous as the emphasis on basic health was, however, it did become a central tenet in modern midwifery, which reestablished itself in 1931 with the opening of the Lobenstine Midwifery Clinic, an outgrowth of the Maternity Center Association. At the clinic, nurse-midwives continued to help a mother be healthy so she could have a healthy child, but they also began to attend deliveries. Between 1931 and 1951, 5,765 mothers registered with the clinic.

Eighty-seven percent of them gave birth at home. Their maternal mortalities were less than a third of the national rate; the neonatal death rates about half.[17] But the world did not take notice.

For over thirty years, evidence of the benefits of midwifery accumulated among the invisible poor. The Chicago Maternity Center, which also opened in 1931, served residents of one of "Chicago's ugliest slums." Babies were delivered "in tenement rooms or cottages that lacked indoor plumbing and sometimes even floors." Midwives, who practiced under the supervision of Dr. Beatrice Tucker, recorded birth outcomes that were "eight to ten times safer than those at Cook County Hospital."[18]

The Frontier Nursing Service was meant to assist the poor mountain women of Kentucky. Its nurses and nurse-midwives also attended to basic health matters: They chlorinated wells, gave treatments for hookworm, provided general medical, dental, and surgical services, tuberculosis treatment, and care for trachoma. They also assisted at births and, in 1932, the Metropolitan Life Insurance Company of New York proclaimed: "If such a service were available to women of the country generally, there would be a saving of 10,000 mothers' lives each year in the United States, there would be 30,000 less stillbirths and 30,000 more children alive at the end of the first month of life."[19] But there followed no hue and cry for the expansion of midwifery. There was no interest shown in understanding its principles.

From that time to this, midwives have proved themselves in the most socially and economically depressed settings. Among migrant farmworkers, among Mexican women who make their way across the border to have their babies, among Native Americans, among urban teenagers, among women of color, again and again and again among the rural poor. Each time midwives moved in, maternal and infant mortality dropped dramatically. But the public's opinion of midwifery did not budge.

In the early sixties, for one last example, a pilot project was run in rural Madera County, California. Midwives began assisting migrant farmworking women who had had no prenatal care. "During the first 18 months of the project, the Madera County . . . neonatal mortality rate dropped from 23.5 per 1,000 births to 10.3 per 1,000 births."[20] Shortly thereafter, the California Medical Society opposed the legalization of nurse-midwifery in that state.

Given this history, we might say that today's public does not accept midwives' perceptions of birth because classism and sexism have gotten in the way. We might even blame doctors—who have tended to be both wealthy and male—for the perpetuation of prejudice. Obviously, this is not entirely inappropriate. The nastiness of the early campaign against midwives has survived inexplicably and cruelly. It is appalling to open the 1983 edition of Danforth's *Obstetrics,* a major text, and observe how it denigrates midwives. Figure 1-1, the first illustration in the book—full page at that—shows a fat, filthy woman with a large, loose-hanging lower lip. The caption reads, "Caricature of a 'midwife going to labor'; holding in her right hand a lamp and in her left a flask of alcoholic refreshment, traditional accoutrements of midwives in the eighteenth and nineteenth centuries." Disbelieving, one looks for the text to correct the impression and does find, a page or so later, buried in the small print of the text, that the type of midwife pictured in Figure 1-1 has had an "unlamented" passing and that there is a "growing corps of well trained nurse-midwives,"[21] but these women are not pictured.

Quite naturally provoked by such misrepresentations, midwives and birth reformers in the last twenty years have engaged in a counteroffensive against overt and covert expressions of hostility toward their profession and its claims about birth. Some have loudly pronounced that doctors "took birth away from women" and that medicine "robbed women of their confidence in their capacity to give birth." They said that male doctors drove women midwives out of business and sacrificed poor urban and rural women on the altar of scientific experimentation and obstetrical education.

Unfortunately, the outcries also imply that midwives and their birth-reforming allies are antimedicine and antiscience, which has done them a disservice. It has diminished the likelihood that their view of birth will be given serious consideration. The language of combat, originating in old wounds and brought to crisis by a growing perception that women in general and midwives in particular were not gaining respect, may have been both necessary and inevitable, but it has not been helpful in conveying an image of midwives as having a keen concern with medical facts. The great American public, not being privy to the history of the conflict, heard midwives charging that medical doctors were hurting women, and they had trouble believing them.

The contentiousness obscured the primary issue. For even if we stipulate that the midwives were right and that their emphasis on good health leading to good birth is correct; even if we agree that women ought, by rights, to be respected; even if we give the midwives their outstanding statistics among the misbegotten, how are we to make a judgment about the quality of their proofs? The midwives showed that they could deliver babies very successfully under the worst of circumstances, but they did not, in fact, put forward the necessary scientific explanations for the success of the births they attended. The absence of evidence gave the medical establishment reason to avoid listening and it gave women carrying babies very little hope that birth might not be a "great emergency."

It left the general public to wonder—if they thought about the subject at all—whether all the midwives' carryings-on about justice and equality were but vague and unprovable claims about the efficacy of birth.[22]

Hindsight

As emotionally provocative and historically determinative as these issues of doctor/midwife, male/female, rich/poor may be, they do not tell us whether the confidence we placed in the opinions of medical science was appropriate. Was birth as dangerous an undertaking as physicians perceived it to be?

To answer, we have to think for a moment about the methods of science and especially how they influence discovery. In particular, we should examine the fact that science, in order to produce universally verifiable information about phenomena, must impose discipline and that such discipline requires the systematic elimination of variables in the phenomena to be studied.

If one wants to know, for example, whether the color of fur has any influence on the length of labor in rats, one must find a batch of brown rats and a batch of white rats of the same variety, put them in identical cages, with identical newspaper shreds on their floors,

and with identical lighting and temperature conditions. Having eliminated as many variables as possible, one can observe the length of
labor in white and brown rats, compare the results, and conclude
that fur color has no bearing on length of labor.

While this method works well in certain investigations, it is insufficient to others. If, for example, one wants to measure the effect of
Pitocin, the labor-stimulating drug, on the length of labor in rats, one
must introduce the control group. One set of rats (same cages, same
newspaper bits) would labor with Pitocin; another set (same cage,
same newspaper bits) would be the control group and labor without
Pitocin. The second group, that is, is to be left entirely alone. Their
undisturbed labor is necessary to prove that Pitocin and not some
other factor is affecting the length of labor in the rats.

This is the sort of experiment, the control group kind, that one
investigator, Niles Newton, used in 1966 to determine whether the
length of labor was affected by the disturbance of labor. She set out
her rats/rats in their cages/cages. When they began to labor, she
disturbed one group—picking them up, setting them down, moving
them from cage to bowl, that sort of thing. The other group she left
in peace. Thus she found that the disturbed rats took longer to
discharge their young than the ones left alone. She also observed that
the disturbed rats had more dead young than the ones left alone.

Newton's experiment creates some imponderable experimental
problems. It makes us think about the universe of environmental
factors that *might* influence a labor—the amount of light in the
room, its temperature, the feel of newspaper on the rats' feet, the
aroma of ink, the kind of metal in the cage, the effect of caging,
the isolation of the parturient rat and so on. Most difficult, however,
it teaches us that it may be impossible to have a true control group
in birth, for there was no way that Newton might observe the rat
without disturbing the rat. The minute she lifted the log in the
woodpile and peered down at the rat nesting there, she would be
disturbing the rat and, presumably, altering the course of its labor.

Keeping these considerations in mind, we look at the scientific
environment in which obstetricians and midwives have practiced.
We remember, for example, that childbirth was to be made more
scientific and more medical by having women move into the hospital

to give birth. We have mentioned one advantage of this arrangement: Students could better learn about birth by practicing on real women. Another, more pertinent, advantage: In the hospital, science could eliminate variables.

In this spirit (if without specific intent), the laboring woman was reduced to a parturient body. She was stripped, scrubbed, smocked, and placed in a hospital bed. The ambient temperature was made relatively consistent, lighting patterns standard, and human influences—family members, for example—removed. By the time a woman was taken to the delivery room (we refer to the first half of the century), variables were even further reduced. The birthing woman was personally extinguished by drugs and her extraneous body parts were covered. We had the rat, not only laboring in the cage, but also drugged and bound.

In light of Newton's later experiment, the scientific errors are evident. If a simple environmental factor like disturbance influences the length and outcome of labor, then what about all the other factors—physical and social—that were present in the early hospital births: unsettlements brought on by race, class, education, architecture, food, isolation, fear, and loss of physical freedom, to name a few. Being scientific, we would have to ask how each of these variables might affect the progress of labor. Ultimately, we would have to ask whether the medical model, which appeared to be so controlled, so free of variables, didn't, in fact, introduce them?

From this perspective, we can hypothesize that medicine may have distorted the very process it was attempting to observe. The experiment itself—medically managed birthing—could be the pathologic agent; it might cause birth to go awry. Indeed, when we review the findings of the early obstetrical researcher, it appears that it might be so. Dr. DeLee wrote in that first volume of the *Journal of Obstetrics and Gynecology* that birth was a pathologic process and, under the circumstances, DeLee could well have been right.

Partly right, that is. Surrounded by the laboratory, DeLee did not factor in its environmental influences. He and others let scientific discipline slide; they failed to keep the experimental conditions in mind. Had DeLee said, "Early twentieth century American hospital birth is pathologic," he would have been correct. But DeLee leaped

carelessly from the particular to the general. He said: Birth is pathologic.

So, while it's been fashionable for some to sneer at Joseph DeLee
for his sexism—teacakes and all—that may be doing him a disservice. His poor opinion of the women's birthing bodies may not have
been due to the overlay of sexual prejudice upon fact, but upon two
major scientific errors. He and his colleagues (1) neglected to establish a control group and (2) wantonly extrapolated from the particular to the general.[1]

Had midwives been permitted into the scientific academy, chances
are good that they would have made similar errors, the fever for
discovery running so high and the reasons to hope being so palpable.
But class and sex kept midwives outside and, by this happenstance,
they observed birth in a relatively natural state. Quite unintentionally, they were the keepers of the control group.

Which is not to say that midwives were uninfluenced by science.
They too eliminated nonspecific birth factors. And while they may
have been acting more out of goodwill than out of scientific purity,
their inoculation programs and their basic health campaigns among
the poor had the effect of removing a vast range of non–birth specific
problems in parturition, all of which gave them a better opportunity
to observe birth in its original form.

In a different laboratory—the home—they drew different conclusions about the process of birth. Midwives saw that some women
labored a long time and still had healthy babies, they saw that labor
stopped in some women, then started up again by itself; they saw
young, old, primip, and multigravid (more than one pregnancy)
women give birth effectively; they realized that many a baby in a
breech position could find his own way.

To be sure, midwives in the first half of this century would not
have attributed their success to "environmental factors" any more
than doctors thought of ascribing their "failures" to the same (although Dr. Tucker guessed that women birthing at home in Chicago
tenements were doing better because they were not alone and frightened; although doctors were aware of the environmental sources of

puerperal fever in the hospital). All midwives knew was that a woman left alone felt more pain than a woman who had someone with her. They knew that a frightened woman had more difficulties at birth. And they knew that birth rewards patience.

They couldn't and didn't prove much. They didn't inaugurate major studies to compare home to hospital births. They assembled no control groups of their own. They did not systematically isolate women. They did not hire researchers to compare the value of doing something to the value of doing nothing. Notably, they did not publish in journals. Midwives went out, they assisted, they were assured by their statistics, and they asserted that birth was not as pathologic as medicine perceived it to be.

Which is to say that midwifery was a way of perceiving and assisting birth that was waiting for proof. Midwives, cast by history into a laboratory that precluded much intervention, took hold of a method of birthing that worked well in that setting and kept it alive. And while they could describe some of the components that seemed to be present in easy births, they could not track precisely from cause to effect.

We think about public image. We note that obstetricians dressed in white, which made them appear to be dispassionate, and that midwives threw their sweaters on, which made them look soft and fuzzy. We note that obstetricians worked in angular, visually antiseptic environments that created an illusion of objectivity and that midwives worked in the chaotic, scientifically unmanageable home. We note that obstetricians adopted the cautious language and analytic customs of science while midwives talked like ordinary people and followed the older, less well-regarded pragmatic tradition.

True, obstetricians reported that birth is generally pathologic, which would seem to be an unattractive message. Midwives spoke more favorably of the process. But when all is said and done, who could have believed them? Women had been dying in those horrendous numbers: How suddenly could it be possible for birth to be safe?

It was never an even race. Medical science, not midwives, delivered the dramatic miracles of the century. The scientists may have erred along the way, they may yet be in error, but they have created, to an extent we could not have imagined at the beginning of the century, a body of knowledge and expertise that makes our imaginations run wild. It is not difficult to understand why our confidence in their judgment has been as great as it has. Neither is it difficult to understand why, under the historical circumstances, women have been unable to develop much confidence in their birthing bodies.

Remembering:
What Mother Told Us

I F BIRTH were just about science, this book would never have needed to be written. Midwives and doctors would have compared their observations about birth, experimented to determine the validity of contested findings, revised their practices, and American women today would not have to figure out for themselves who or what to believe about their bodies at birth. But birth is human and historical and cultural and so it is only today that such exchanges are beginning to take place.

If birth were just about science, then women would have understood by now that good health generally means strong, healthy birth and that meddling can interfere with outcome. But birth is human and alive and responsive. The way women think about it comes not only from professionals but from their mothers, the ones who've given birth before them.

The stories that mothers tell their daughters about birth have been shaped by nearly a century of experience in hospital birth. Here's what today's women say they learned:

> "We never talked much about those things in my family."

> "I know my mother was terrified of childbirth . . . but she never said anything."

> "It seems that information just sort of filtered in . . . in whispers, with some giggles—some information rather revolting, some unbelievable. I was not prepared for the physical side of childbirth when my still-born son arrived. . . . I know my mother never told me anything."

> "Nothing much. . . . It was something you had to go through. There was nothing you could do about it."

> "I think with my brothers she was out completely."

> "My mother never talked about birth very much."

> "My mother never said anything."

We have silent grandmothers today. Older women without birth stories. Women without life-giving poetry. Themes, rich with pattern and variation of pattern, do not lap from a mother's experience into her daughter's imagination. The first questions: Where did I come from? How did I get here? How was I born? What was birth like for you? Essential questions about life and womanhood go unanswered. The mothers of today's mothers, the traditional keepers of the tales that are a woman's legacy, are mute. It seems as if birth, like an orphan, had been disconnected from its source.

Women today take for granted the absence of the word. They must think it is the way life is, this having mothers who cannot describe what it's like for the human female to bud, break, and bear fruit. Perhaps they think all young mothers have done without, not knowing that in other times the traditions of birth simmered, making the very aroma of women's lives, that women tended each other in their homes and huts, chanting or singing hymns, preparing broths and hot cloths, oiling, massaging, whispering, giving instruction; that they slept by one another's beds in chairs, prepared food, consulted in kitchens, entangled arms and legs, washed the living, dressed and buried the dead; that the dramas of birth staked women's lives and lore unfurled from them.

Today's grandmothers are silent. How do we account for it? For even though they gave birth in hospitals, they should have stories of some kind—even disheartening ones. One has to wonder what kind of women these were, the mothers of today's mothers, that they have no birth stories to tell. Did they discount themselves so much that the experience of birth seemed not to have happened to them? Were they so enthralled with medicine that they simply rolled over and let physicians and the hospitals have their way? Did they not have their heads about them at all?

These are legitimate possibilities, considering the generation of women we inquire about. Today's grandmothers, the women of the fifties, the women of the *Feminine Mystique,* after all, are the ones from whom we took flight as twentieth-century feminists. They were the ones, Betty Friedan told us in 1963, who were taught that domesticity equaled fulfillment and who believed, in the postdestruction shadow of World War II, that of all things, nests must be relined. At least they seemed to have thrown themselves into having babies and making homes where repetitious domestic work made them bored, frustrated, depressed, and inexplicably tired. When they found themselves miserable, as they often did, they dutifully went to therapists who told them that something was wrong with their femininity. If they were unfulfilled by housework, there must be something askew in them. " 'Normal' femininity is achieved," Friedan wrote, explaining the philosophy of the time, " . . . insofar as the woman finally renounces all active goals of her own, all her own 'originality.' "[1]

So these women, today's grandmothers, banged away, like mechanics on the bent fenders of mass-produced cars, on the parts of themselves that didn't follow the pattern of 'normal' femininity. They went to physicians who, applying a chemical therapy, tranquilized them so they would not have to feel the curse of their frustrated potential. They treated themselves, as oppressed people have always done, with the drugs at hand—Librium, Valium, and alcohol.

What Friedan doesn't emphasize, what feminists have understated, and what today's young women often overlook, however, is that those same women, in that same pattern of oppression, were also obliterated and rearranged in childbirth. They entered the hospital and they were put out. They were chemically deterred from experiencing the original female experience. Following medical science, they missed the primary experience of birth.

When we consider the fact that their motherhood was supposed to be the very reason for their existence, this is a considerable paradox. Why did they allow it? Why were they speechless? And, more pertinent, why have their daughters, who have exhaustively discussed their mothers' social, political, economic, and artistic silence, barely mentioned the equally deafening silence about birth?

Their mothers' lives, after all, prompted the feminist revolution of this century. The oppression their mothers endured enraged women and made them fight for dignity. It has been the duty of this generation to accuse its predecessors and tear themselves away, in their mothers' names, for themselves and for their sisters and daughters. To the degree that a woman's life is freer and fuller than her mother's, she considers herself advanced. And women have been successful in meeting their historical assignment. Generally speaking, women have given up the ghettoed aspect of suburban life. Few women today would say that they should be self-abnegating. Few believe that they, like Eve, shouldn't be curious about and active in life beyond the patio-garden.

But today's women, like Leslie, following their mothers' pattern, are relatively silent about their births. They rarely accuse their mothers of having been too passive in childbirth. They do not raise questions about their birth behavior. And so we must assume that some workable truth endures; we must assume that there was then, and that there continues to be now, some solid, underlying reason for an obliterative choice.

If we are to understand the silence of women today, we may need to think once more about the generations of women who preceded them and look more closely at how they experienced their births. One more time, sort through their bureau drawers, look at the family photograph albums, throw our imaginations around the conditions that framed the lives of women during this last, transforming century. Think why birth was missing.

Absolute Powerlessness

We know now that labor is prolonged and birth pain augmented by fear and anxiety. Since feelings of fear and anxiety are provoked by powerlessness, there can be no doubt that the women who went into the hospital to save themselves and their babies endured more difficult and more painful labors than they would have had at home, simply because they were in an unfamiliar environment. Indeed, the more the well-intended doctors poked, prodded, directed, and isolated women, the more pain relief was needed. The doctors, sensitive to women's suffering, unable to provide the constant human companionship that might ease it, searched for better, more effective artificial pain relievers.

In 1914, they hit upon scopolamine. Scopolamine, an amnesic, was used in combination with morphine to produce what was called Twilight Sleep, and it appeared to solve all the problems of birth. It did not suppress a woman as ether and chloroform did. Where those drugs caused her to become dead weight, a nonpushing body, Twilight Sleep seemed to liberate a woman's animal self. Its amnesic component separated her from her body, which could writhe, toss, even feel pain, but all outside her recognizance. Although they sometimes had to put her in a high-sided, canvas-walled crib to keep her from tossing herself out of bed or "wandering aimlessly" on the labor floor, although they might have had to tie her arms and legs down to keep her from doing damage to herself, her body did move during labor. She could hear the doctor, she did as he bid, she pushed. They told her that she would awaken "so free from fatigue or soreness that she could leave her bed at once and care for her own baby."[2]

Twilight Sleep appeared to provide the best of all possible worlds. It was a return to "more physiological birth" without the return to pain—a point not lost on women. "Take up the battle for painless childbirth," one of many female journalists urged her readers. "Fight not only for yourselves, but fight for your . . . sex."[3] Women with substantial reputations—"new women," crusading women, women physicians—organized the National Twilight Sleep Association and sponsored rallies in department store aisles so that ordinary women would hear about the drug that would ease a woman through her trial. Energetically, they dispersed the reports that scopolamine meant less heart strain, fewer cervical lacerations, fewer forceps deliveries, and better milk secretions. It was said to be the dawning of a new age in childbirth.

Of course there were the usual detractors: professionals who questioned the wisdom of interfering unnecessarily with a healthy process and who made the tired complaint that Twilight Sleep, like any other suppressant drugs, compromised newborn respiration. But the women, undaunted, "demanded their traditional right to decide how they would have their children. . . . [They] wanted to control their own births by choosing to go to sleep. . . . They were demanding, as women had always demanded . . . their right to control their own birthing experiences."[4]

It took some time to discover all the effects of Twilight Sleep. At first, no one realized that it not only put women out of their minds, but that it also distorted them.

> I can't remember much about the actual labor except that they were giving me Twilight Sleep. . . . I remember nothing about the delivery. . . . I know I had an episiotomy and when I awakened I was in my room and, of course, I was feeling high. You always do after a birth. I went to call my mother and my first clue as to how deadly that stuff was, was that I couldn't see to dial the phone and then . . . I was supposed to rest and I remember laying in bed and looking at those horrible draperies . . . sort of tan and those things were breathing.[5]

It could lead to overdrugging:

> On admission, patients were given 3 ccs of Seconal IV [intravenous], 75 of Demerol, 25 of Phenergen, 1/150th of scopolamine, followed in a half an hour by 1/100th of scopolamine, followed in half an hour by 1/100th of scopolamine. I would get these women in who were excited, happy to be in labor or terrified to be in labor . . . within an hour they were sound asleep and I would have to watch their toes . . . to know that they were ready to deliver.[6]

And it displaced women. This drug, elected by vast numbers of American women over several decades, succeeded by stealth where the most ambitious sexists might fear to go.

Now in her seventies, Jacqueline Page is a tiny regent of rebellion. Her bronzed hair is swept up to coronal heights. Her sitting room is set with carefully collected, highly polished brass and copper antiques. She has no tolerance for crass consumerism and the ungracious pace of American life. She not only knows her own mind, but acquaints others with it.

In 1937 she was pregnant with her son Mike. Since Jac has the body of a lark, her doctor was concerned about the baby's size. He told her that her pelvic measurements were "almost juvenile," prescribed a cautious diet, and decided finally to induce her labor before her son lost all sense of proportion (which he has since done from time to time).

He [the doctor] explained that when the induced labor began . . . a rectal anesthetic by enema would be employed. I objected and said, "But how will I know what is happening and how can I help my baby to be born?" He replied, "You will know what is happening and you will follow my instructions all the way but you won't remember a thing."

After the induced labor began, things moved along in a natural way and soon the anesthetic was given and I passed serenely into oblivion. Fourteen hours later I saw faces through a fog and heard voices from a distance saying, "Too big, too big" and "My God . . . he's enormous!" Then blackout.

I learned later that although a section had been avoided, some tearing had occurred in bringing forth a nine-and-a-half pounder and multiple stitches were required, and forceps were also necessary, although they left the child unmarked.

The following day I said to my good doctor, "Now tell me how I helped my son to be born. I remember absolutely nothing." He pulled a chair close to my bed and placed his hand over mine.

"It's like amnesia," he said. "The anesthetic induced forgetfulness . . . you were aware of everything but you cannot remember. You were very brave and you worked very hard but you don't remember now. Does that disturb you?"

His eyes searched mine, concerned.

I assured him that it did not as long as my baby was healthy and sound and that I had done my best.[7]

Women give birth in the best way they can. Their most urgent need, their greatest responsibility, is to get that life out from under their ribs and into their arms without losing it during the passage. If that means personal obliteration, so be it. If it means placing control in the hands of another person, then it will be done. If it means diminishing independence, then accommodate, submit, rearrange.

The initial frenzy of enthusiasm for scopolamine did not last long. When one its leading proponents, a Mrs. Francis X. Carmody, died in childbirth in 1915, a more moderate view of the drug emerged. Nevertheless, it continued to be used into the sixties and its impact—the idea of painless childbirth—has remained a powerful force in American childbirth. Drugs, like Demerol and epidurals and spinals, gradually replaced it.

But Twilight Sleep has a half-life in our psyches. It effectively sealed a generation of women off from the experience of power and capability at birth. Over time, it distorted women's expectations of what they are capable of so that today, women have no way to know what they miss. It and all the other drugs that have been employed for the last century and a half patterned our minds and made us think that half a birth is a whole birth and that a whole birth is a twist of nature.

"Almost a freak," the grandmother said, sitting in her New York apartment, certain of the word she chose to describe her son's late fifties birth. "There was no time for any anesthesia so it was very quick and painful and exhilarating. Screaming one minute, laughing the next, and I felt terrific afterward because there was no time for any anesthesia. . . . I felt very close to euphoria, a mystic, kind of a religious experience, but . . . strictly a freak."[8]

Women were liberating themselves from the lethal aspects of childbirth when they chose medical care. A side effect was that their minds and spirits were quenched. The hearth fires were put out; reproductive power was forgotten, the oral record silenced. Pregnant women today, preparing for the eternally returning experience of birth, listen for the voices inscribed in their minds during childhood.

They hear nothing. Their hearts being ignorant, they must write their births out of their heads. "Orphans," Carl Becker has written of those who have lived in the scientific centuries following the Enlightenment, "abandoned in the cosmos."

Because of our interest in saving our children's lives, we lost the legacy of childbirth. As we did, we sealed ourselves off from knowledge of our capacities, and thus we came to believe that physicians must shore up birth. Without personal knowledge of the power that comes to us unbidden during birth, we came to believe that it did not exist. Without it, we believed we were inadequate to the task. And we were correct. Without that visiting power, we are.

Remembering:
The Inner Legacy

When I, Sheryl, first met Penny in the early seventies, she was smoking brown cigarettes, refusing to make coffee, and celebrating the fact that she'd beaten a father of three out of a job. A few years thereafter, I remember her shoving a broken-spirited me down on the couch and, in a noble effort to convince me of my invincibility, made me sing along to Helen Reddy's Greatest Hit: "I am woman, hear me roar."

We have both acted out many of the feminist dramas of the time. We were born in the eclipse years of the *Feminine Mystique* and we have been no less confused, destroyed, buoyed, irritated, thrilled, and frightened than most other women by the intense effort that we have made to be heard and respected. The feminist factor has been part of our lives.

We mention this because we want to take advantage of the feminist axiom that the "personal is the political" or, as we alter it here, the "personal is the cultural." Our lives, feminists discovered, are one of our best resources. They can help us gain insight into the inner and common dynamics of women's experience.

Penny and I have each been shaped by twentieth-century birth. From giving birth, I acquired guilt and shame; from watching lifeless women give birth, Penny learned about the dynamics of contempt for women. Our experiences seem relevant to our effort to understand why women think poorly of their birthing selves. If the way women give birth induces shame in them, as it did with me; if the way women birth makes observers think less of them, as Penny saw that it did, then it is possible that medicalized birth, discovered by the mothers of this century, insidiously perpetuates itself in women's low evaluation of themselves.

Original Sin

My sons were born in 1962 and 1964. I knew that the *Feminine Mystique* had come out in the year between their births, but I didn't read it then. In spite of the following account of my good-girl births, I was worried about being too independent-minded for my own good, and I wanted to quell my propensities as much as possible. I had those babies to think of.

More to the point, I first became pregnant when I was young—barely into my twenties—and, due to abundant California sunshine and the innumerable salads that were a way of life in that state, shamelessly healthy. It's true, I wasn't particularly well prepared for birth. My sex education had actually started when an older neighbor girl showed me her blood, but officially it came from the often-cited movie put out by Kotex. As a billboard fifties' child—that is, white and middle class—I sat in the community room of a white, Protestant church in suburbia, wearing my Girl Scout uniform, flashing my badges for basket weaving and home nurse, and watched butterflies flitting about boxes of "sanitary" napkins. Hearing about this, my mother handed me a slim, clinical volume that described the impregnating act which, also typically, quite took me aback.

I don't remember Mom telling me much about birth except that my big brother's head was dangerously big, that I was just about born in the toilet (which she thought gave early evidence of my later penchant for inappropriate behavior and which I eventually learned is about as healthy a birth as an infant can come by), and that my younger brothers, the twins—well, it happened so fast you couldn't really discuss it.

That and marital sex sums up what I knew about reproduction. When I was pregnant, I read a couple of books, but not too many were written then about how to give birth. We concentrated on baby care in those days and my husband and I went to Red Cross classes where we diapered and bathed dolly. If it hadn't been for my neighbor, Jeannie Fruzyna, who had her first baby three months before I was due, I wouldn't have known that you always had a spinal or an epidural. She said it hurt when they gave you the shot, but that didn't put me off. I had played a lot of tag football growing up with three brothers and I figured I could manage a needle in my back. What perplexed me was how such a big thing as a baby could get out of such a small hole.

Girls like me did what our doctors said. So, when my doctor examined me on my due date and said that I would have my baby that night and that he did not care to get up in the middle of it, nor did he wish to miss the barbeque dinner he had planned with his wife, I courteously replied that I could see his interests. We met at the hospital at four in the afternoon; he stayed long enough to get an induction started and then, I guess, he went home to drip liquid fire-starter on his briquets. I told him I would do my best not to disrupt his dinner.

When the anesthesiologist came in later, I obediently offered him my spine. At 8:18, a mere four hours after I arrived at the hospital and just a half an hour after the doctor returned, my husband and I watched, nonplussed and ecstatic, as a real live boy baby was pulled out of me. Our eyes followed him while they fussed with him at a faraway table and then carried him out of the delivery room.

The doctor, meanwhile, was sewing the requisite episiotomy, which I afterward thought of as a painful but necessary proof of my passage into motherhood. I felt it was a woman's secret badge, comparable in my imagination to circumcision rituals for young boys who grew up in jungles. I sat stoically and proudly on pillows for a couple of weeks and my ruddy-faced, immaculate, and miraculous son Chuckie nursed exuberantly.

My second pregnancy was as healthy as the first. While it ran its course, Chuckie and I played like puppies—I hadn't really used up my own childhood—we went for walks, read picture books, stacked blocks, imitated animals, cooked dinner, cleaned house, got a room ready for the new baby, and went to the airport the night before my due date to pick up my mother.

I don't remember having Pitocin with Mike, but I do remember contractions rolling over me like axe-carrying thunderheads and the arrival of the anesthetist, who screwed the needle into my spine and pumped a little juice into my system. I waited trustingly for the pain to halt and when it didn't, the anesthetist squeezed in more juice, pinched my skin, and poked my bones. I felt it all. I suspect now that my shamelessly healthy body was ignoring the pitiful attempts of drugs to influence it, but at the time I was concentrating on the upcoming episiotomy. I knew the doctor cut deep and I wasn't interested in enduring the perineal equivalent of amputation without benefit of anesthesia. I asked for more juice. On the way to the delivery room, the anesthetist and I joked cavalierly about how stubborn the pain was. What I remember from the birth is that the doctor swore at the nurses and that he flashed forceps.

In those days, in that town, "they" didn't bring your baby until the next day. I remember the receiving blanket was folded over Mikie's face when the nurse put him next to me and it wasn't until the two of us were alone that I lifted the tip of the blanket back and saw that my new baby's face was puffed and pale like an old alcoholic's and that his temples were swollen, black and blue.

I sucked in my breath and when I breathed out I seemed to be on some foul and swampy shore. What kind of an issue was this? Clawed, bloated, and sludgy the baby was, as if he'd come up through slimy grasses and mud. Weighted, thick, and dull. He would never laugh, this child. He would not jump in his crib. I dared not think myself of what debris-ridden, tangled thoughts might one day come to him. What thing had I done? What sin had I committed? How could such a fen-ish baby be born to a well-behaved young woman who tried so hard? I wanted to suck him back inside of me where he'd been safe and back to a time when we'd both been innocent.

Mikie wouldn't open his eyes. It seemed to me that he was trying, but his lids wouldn't budge. I stroked his cheek, spoke to him, introduced myself, cajoled him, offered him my breast, stroked his head, held his hand. He remained thick and unresponsive. I teased his mouth with my nipple. Nothing. With killing indifference, his face stayed dull. I knew he was going to die and I thought the nurse would never come and take him away and let me cry, which I did, sickened by my inability to take care of him, grieving for the lifelessness which, it seemed, I had somehow caused.

By the time our three-day hospital stay was about up, things had improved. Not only had Mike faintly nursed, not only were his bruises turning a reassuring yellow, but I had recovered somewhat from the birth, refound my footing, reclaimed my youthful sense of invincibility, and was confident that I could love him into life. That was when the nurse, who was dressing him for departure, said, "I'm sorry to have to send you home with this baby. He's kept us very busy in the nursery."

And I was thrown back again. To what had been wrong. To what was really wrong with him. My fault.

"What do you mean?"

"Oh nothing. But he's kept us busy."

Mikie had been crying was all she would say. Oh, I'd been gossiping with the other women in the wards, opening baby presents, waving through the window at Chuckie, assuming Mikie was sleeping, OK, safe, healing, getting his diapers changed, when in fact, Mikie'd been down the hallway in a plastic bassinette, making siren calls, begging for solace, for arms, for reassurance that he didn't have to do this, this being alive, on his own. The nerve, not telling me, I thought, in passing; but unloosed upon that, submerging it, was: Why hadn't I found out? Why hadn't I taken up vigil at the nursery window automatically, beaten on the glass when he cried, kicked them out of the way, claimed him, held him, rocked him, soothed him: I grabbed Mikie from the nurse, pulled him to me, and gritted my teeth for the long journey by wheelchair, out the front door of the hospital and to the car. I would make him, absolutely *make him* thrive.

Mike was twenty years old and decidedly life-prone when I first went out with Penny to Amish home births. I must have held fifteen or so newborns in my arms, watching their faces pink up, seeing the clear wonder in their eyes, before it hit me that it hadn't been my fault, that Mikie's eyes hadn't been sludged shut because of something wrong with my body, but because of the drugs they'd given him; that my baby hadn't been able to bring himself to nurse not because of something wrong with my breast, but because he was too hung over; and that he hadn't squalled in the nursery because he had a difficult temperament but because he had splitting headache from the clamp of those forceps.

My sons' first impression of life on earth was of assault and isolation, and that was wrong. There had been joy imminent and the hospital had made grief; there had been fecundity present and they had made sterility; there had been fullness waiting and they had made scarcity. There had been confirmation of health at hand, and they had made us both feel weak.

When I saw those babies born at home, I gave up the feeling that there had been something wrong with my body at Mike's birth. But I quickly replaced one guilt with another: I should have been smarter, I should have been less naive, I should have demanded rooming-in, I should have found out about natural childbirth—even though, considering when I lived, I would have had to have invented it myself.

The Multiplication of Sin

An anthropologist writes that "if the infant is born malformed or ill, many societies will consider the parents at fault for having failed to follow prescribed pregnancy patterns. Thus many other parents as well as many contemporary American parents are felt to be somehow accountable for the welfare and normal development of the fetus."[1]

Problems with pregnancy and birth, in other words, apparently devolve back onto the parent, and most particularly, the mother. We follow the "prescribed pregnancy patterns," thinking we are doing our best and that we should therefore be approved by our family and friends. If those prescribed pregnancy patterns result in damage, however, it feels not like their fault, but ours. It's damned if you do, damned if you don't. If you break the rules to get a better birth, you expose yourselves to criticism from your loved ones; if you don't break them and your children suffer, you shoulder the agonizing aftermath.

It took me a long time to figure this out. First I had to admit that I had not invented American birth style in 1964, which was hard because it required me to admit that I wasn't the independent agent I had feared myself to be in those years. In fact, I'd been more like a Chevrolet, stamped out by the culture I was raised in. As you might discern from what I have written, my ego resisted this insight.

Even with the benefit of some humility, however, I knew that I kept the guilt and that I always would. I think it's because pregnancy, birth, and early baby care are so irrefutably personal. In the end, a mother and child, or primary parent and child, are alone and must work out how to survive together. But the parent, being older, feels the weight of the responsibility, which is like being a god. Without the powers.

I've never objected to this distortion, this feeling that I was totally responsible for my children's lives. Nature must have invented it, I thought then and think now: Otherwise we might not protect our children with our lives. Nevertheless it had taken taken me twenty years to see who had made what happen at Mike's birth and to begin to wonder why I had assumed all the responsibility when, in fact, it was more properly shared. Why hadn't it occurred to me to criticize the hospital system rather than my body?

Familiar Guilt

Sheila Kitzinger is best known for her contributions to the understanding of the psychosexual aspects of childbirth. One afternoon in 1987, I was in her living room with a hundred women from around the world to discuss the subject. Sitting in chairs, on the arms of chairs, on the floors, and leaning up against the ancient doorframes of Sheila's manor house near Oxford, England, we discussed all the gooey, slippery, wet, and bulging aspects of pregnancy and birth and how they were perceived by women from different places.

Into this sometimes saucy, sometimes moving talk, she threw in a comment about how she and two of her daughters, who worked in Rape Crisis and Incest Survivor Services, had observed a similarity between the reactions of women who were raped and those who had been obstetrically abused. No one at the workshop pursued the comment, which I thought was interesting in itself, so I wrote her later to find out what she was referring to.

The three of them, she responded, had sorted out the "similarity of the rape trauma syndrome with women's feelings, behavior and language following a violent birth with invasive obstetric procedures." She illustrated how the two situations are similarly set up. In incest, for example, the father often blames the daughter for his crime. "When a girl resists [incestuous] rape the father often becomes abusive and calls her a 'slut' and 'whore.' He tells her she is 'selfish' for not wanting sex with him." Thus she assumes the responsibility for the violation. In childbirth, blame is similarly placed on the woman: "When a woman resists an invasive obstetric procedure, she may also be reviled and told she is 'selfish,' concerned only with her own emotions and even be accused of not caring whether she kills her baby."

Having been instructed by the reigning authorities that she is bad and they are good, she can only assume that any ensuing damage is her fault. After rape, women characteristically "present themselves as worthless and deserving of punishment because there is something wrong with *them.*" They criticize themselves: " 'It was really all my fault.' They feel intense guilt: 'I asked for it. I shouldn't have walked across the park that night'; 'I was a little flirt, daddy couldn't help it'; 'I'm responsible for breaking up a happy family.' "

The same self-accusatory language is used by women who have had difficulty at birth. "Women tended to believe that when an epidural did not work it must be their fault, because they were too fat, did not lie still enough, or had a 'funny' spine." Or women will say, " 'I didn't push hard enough'; I should have practised my breathing more.' "[2]

It doesn't take a lot of analysis to see why women in either situation—first put down and then invaded—would absorb shame. Typically, in rape, they turn it inward and "suffer depression. . . . They experience anger which is turned in on to themselves." Having been raped myself, having several friends who have been raped, I was not unfamiliar with the syndrome Sheila and her daughters describe. We all blamed ourselves. For many of us, it's such a powerful violation it brings up all the sexual shame we have accumulated in our lives. It slugs us and, at first, we can't see our way clear to accuse the perpetrator. It is only later, as we tell our story over and over, weeding out the underlying sources of shame, that we learn that we didn't deserve the abuse, that there really are some destructive men in the world, and that they might act on us—regardless of our personal qualities.

But we are not yet in the habit of sorting through our births this way, of separating the necessary from the unnecessary invasions. It may be a next step, one that will follow our naming of assault *as* assault. After all, abuse in birth is more subtle: The invaders do not lurk behind bushes, pry open doors, nor throw us to the floor. They hold no knives to our throats. And while some do tie us up, they are not terrible people at all; most of them intend the best. And when they're done, we're not just split open—we have babies and we are thankful. In birth, invasion is not black and white. We feel we cannot complain because everyone seems to have done their level best.

But we would do well to remind ourselves that depression does not cease to be anger "which is turned in on to themselves" simply because it occurs postpartum.

Which recalls the era of the *Feminine Mystique* and how all those women assumed that their unhappiness was their fault. And how, even though we've had a woman's revolution since then and even though we've had an era of birth reform, we are at least as violated in birth as before. Adrienne Rich's chilling chapter, "Hands of Flesh, Hands of Iron" in her 1976 book *Of Woman Born* has not made us rise up and stay there; Suzanne Arms's 1978 *cri de coeur, Immaculate Deception,* did not turn us away from medicalized birth, and Nancy Wainer Cohen and Louis J. Estner's 1983 book, *Silent Knife,* was not followed by a drop in cesarean rates.

These writers' exhortations, eloquent and impassioned as they might be, are weak in proportion to the power of guilt and shame and all the other factors that discourage healthy birth. They fade by proportion; they are usurped by our close-lying and misguided sense of responsibility for the problems of birth. We dare not believe the birth reformers because if we do we must accept that damage was done to us. Much more difficult, we must admit that people we trusted, whom we had to trust, hurt us. And after that, we would have to accept the possibility that our birthing bodies might work.

Afterword

I must add that I gave this chapter to my mother to read in draft. After she finished, she told me the full story of my older, big-headed brother's birth. When she was at term, she said, the doctor had her X-rayed. It was then that she was advised that her baby's head was exceptionally large. No particular plans were made, however, and so she went into labor. After twenty-four hours of it in the hospital, the doctor stopped by. Making no mention of the big head, or of options, he told her that her baby would be born the next day. He went off to get some sleep.

He was right. My brother was delivered the next morning. In the process, however, my mother's interior parts were cut, ruptured, and split. I believe this because she spent a lot of time in the hospital having them repaired when I was growing up. I, as the only daughter, filled in for her, knowing only that there was something wrong with her female parts and wondering if I would inherit the same weaknesses.

When I asked her what she thought about her doctor now, she said she thought he was a nice man. He who had failed to talk with her about the big head once she was in the hospital; he who had not mentioned the case for or against cesarean; he who had let her labor all night against the head and against the belief that it was too big; he who had slept through the ordeal; he who had delivered the baby violently, doing lifetime damage to her body. Nice.

As much as we know about the oppression of women, as much as we learn about the dynamics of victimization, it is a struggle to admit that abuse has been done to us. It requires too much of us. It asks us to contradict our vast, inner resources of shame and, simultaneously, to challenge those who put it there.

For many of us, this asks too much. It is more consistent with our lives to accept the mutilation and the damage. We might spend half a lifetime recovering from birth injuries, but it is difficult for us to consider the possibility that it might be the medical system that has caused them.

Compounding Guilt

Guilt and shame are incurred in a climate of disrespect. Once within us, they often behave greedily, seeking ever more evidence that we are right to think poorly of ourselves. It may be a perversity of our psychological nature that causes this, but it can't be ignored in birth any more than it can be ignored in the rest of our lives. Penny's experience illustrates the dynamics:

Being born in northern Maine, I had no idea that women were supposed to be lesser. To the contrary, I thought all women had muscles, staunch beliefs, and local power. The women I knew sweated; they fought the elements; they felt birth, health, illness, and death between their thumbs and forefingers; they reported to a very strict God.

We didn't need any toy stoves in our house, my mother said, since I was perfectly able to learn to cook on the real one. And then she set me to cleaning house, weeding the garden, and helping in the kitchen. If I forgot that these were chores that others needed me to do, I was sent to my room until I sorted it out. I learned this way—in combination, that is, with the games my mother played with me, the baths she drew for me, and the food she prepared—that I was both dependable and worthy.

Sometimes I lived out on the family farm and sometimes in a small apartment over my father's grocery store. In the town, I have to say, a woman's life did not look as vital as it did in the country. As far as I could tell, my mother's town life consisted of fishing for the forks my brothers and I had thrown down the heat register. So I left my mother's dull rooms upstairs and took myself down below, where I found barrels, racks of brightly colored magazines, and machines that spewed out long links of sausages. With my father as my companion, I made blood-curdling trips to the slaughterhouse and illicit (I sensed) border crossings into Canada. Sometimes Dad stuffed live pigs, head first, into potato barrels, tossed them on the back of the pickup truck, and everyone, including me and the border guards, had to pretend they weren't there. We always succeeded and I thought I could do anything.

I was included in birth. We had a farm in New Hampshire when I was twelve and Dad decided we should have sheep. Having let them frolic in the wrong month of the year, we faced lambing in February. It was snowing and the barn was bitterly cold, but we—that is, me, my mother, my two brothers, and the vet—sprang to. I remember the sober, excited feeling of being in on the myth-sized matters that concerned adults.

Way into the night we were busy building tents over the stalls. We passed tacks, hammers, ropes, and rigging, saying little, because words took time. When the first sheep started huffing and bleating, we ran for the portable space heater and rushed it to the rescue. I remember clinging to my post in the haystack night after night, forcing myself awake, hoping one more lamb would get stuck and that the vet would call me over and ask me to reach inside the sheep's uterus and pull out a stuck lamb. No one else could do that as well as me, with my slender arms. In this way, I became an atypical girl, associating femaleness and birth with power and competence.

It wasn't until I began my nurse's training in St. Louis, Missouri, in 1975 that I began to question my convictions. My experiences there almost put an end to my plan to become a midwife and nearly destroyed my confidence in the integrity of women. I, who had had the impression that medical people comforted and healed, was shocked by the brutality I encountered; I, who believed that women were strong, brave, and active, was deeply disturbed by observing women who were not.

Our introduction to maternity nursing was a film, not of a full-bodied woman at the height of her power pushing a child into the world, but of a near-dead woman, suffering from postpartum hemorrhage. I remember that our teacher had barely introduced the film, let alone maternity nursing, before she shut off the lights and had us watch torrents of red, grainy blood pouring from a comatose woman. As far as I can remember, no one in the film did anything for the woman; the message we took, and I did take it, was that laboring women, lying very still, were always about to die and that there was little we could do about it.

With no palliative words from the teacher, I found myself, scrubbed, gowned, in a delivery room, and at the side of a screaming, writhing woman. Tied with leather straps, carrying on, she wasn't acting like any of the women I identified with. She was nothing more than a frantic, confused animal caught in a snare.

Ignoring her completely was a masked nurse. She had her back turned to the patient and her hands were coolly positioning surgical instruments on a metal tray. As I fumbled with the incongruity, alternately forcing myself to be of a tough, medical mind and rebelling against the indifference I was witnessing, the swinging doors bumped open and an anesthesiologist and an obstetrician entered the room. Without greeting us, the doctor said, "Go," and the anesthesiologist slapped a mask over the woman's nose. She slumped.

The obstetrician nodded to the nurse, who slipped him scissors, which he immediately and generously applied to the woman's lifeless perineum. Feeling dizzy and sick at the sight of retreating flesh and the flow of blood, I fought to find all that internal toughness I prided myself on. To avoid fainting, I shifted my weight.

My new position allowed me to see a dark smear of life grunting toward the woman's splayed vagina. For all the thick and wetness, I was stilled by the approach of life—shunted into eternality—

and I half expected the others in the room to bow their heads. Instead, I saw the doctor's hand, extended by chill-looking forceps, plunge toward the oncoming head. He clamped it hard, dragged the blade up and down, wrenching the woman's flesh in the process. I took every assault in myself. Each one exploded in my groin and pinioned my guts. I was trembling when I saw that the baby's head had landed between the woman's thighs. The doctor tossed the forceps aside. He and the nurse exchanged comments about the weather.

I fixed on the baby's face, which was compacted, puffy, blue, covered with blood and, without question, dead-looking. I knew babies didn't look like magazine photographs at birth, but this was something else again; its face was clumped like stale lard. My mind was shooting to the devastating moment ahead when I, shamelessly unprepared, would speak to the mother of a stillborn child, when the doctor straightened himself, put his hands around the baby's head and dragged a baby girl's body out her mother's wound. With every cell of my body, I silently commanded the infant to jerk, tremble, bubble at the mouth, or flinch a muscle. The doctor nipped the baby up by her ankles, swung her from from her heels and whapped her bottom. Nothing. He slapped her again. It was the third swat that made her whimper.

Of course I could not make sense of it. The doctor and nurse were oblivious; that much was clear. But I told myself that they must know what they were doing whereas I, surely, did not: I was the one who had thought that baby was dead. Besides, the woman *had* been writhing and screaming. What else could they do but put her out? Was it possible that women might not be strong?

I was so upset by what I was seeing that I considered reregistering for an emergency room specialty. But the holidays came and with them, an opportunity to make some money by filling in for some vacationing maternity nurses at the public hospital we were affiliated with.

To be sure, one had to need money to take an assignment at City Hospital, which was located in a neighborhood of drug runners and snipers. The building itself was decomposing and when my nursing school roommate and I walked in, we were greeted by an armed guard, who directed us to maternity, which was decorated with three patched-up Christmas tree ornaments tacked to a bulletin board. The charge nurse sent us to meet our first patient, seventeen-year-old Marie, a girl with a body no more substantial than a dime-store crèche figure.

Nervously, she chattered about her boyfriend, Strawberry, who belonged to a motorcycle gang. She did too, she said, whipping up her gown to show us her tattooed thigh. She wanted to have her baby immediately, she advised us, because she intended to strap it on her back tomorrow and buzz off to a cycle rally. We winced, thinking of the swollen and bruised postpartum bottoms we'd seen, but Marie bewitched us with her enthusiasm and we set about doing everything we could to make her plan work.

Amazing us, she soon began to shudder with wet, dense breaths. Her body heaved with contractions. Her eyes masked over and her knees drew up toward her chin. She tossed her tiny arms behind her knees, and out of her came a coarse rumble, as if bone and muscle had been struck. We lifted her, this charming child/reverberant woman, to a stretcher.

Dr. Arafa, a thatchy-browed man with a laborer's mien and Middle Eastern accent, greeted us from the delivery room door. Noticing that the room was strangely bare of nurses or anesthesiologists, I first rebelled at him and then at a society that distributed resources so inequitably. But Dr. Arafa, who was too imperfect to be frightening, assured us that he was "the best," and when he settled himself between Marie's birdlike thighs and began to explain to us what he was doing, I forgot my complaints. He allowed us to talk to Marie, and he himself called her by name when he asked for her pushes. He did cut her, but for the first time in my experience, I saw a flushed and lively face appear from underneath a pubic bone. It rested there while Dr. Arafa fixed his eyes on Marie's face and asked for one more push, just like the one before. The baby rode out into his hands, wriggled, stretched, and sprang a cry.

It was enough to rekindle my belief. And while few other women at City showed the same mettle as Marie, I saw sparks of it from time to time. I got the first whiff of the idea that an eruption of birth might be in women, waiting to be called out. In fleeting moments, I began to suspect a relationship between respect and birth.

A British-trained midwife asked us to labor-sit with a sallow-skinned, inner-city woman named Patsy. I had already learned that I couldn't compensate for another woman's vacant lots in the few short hours I had with her, but I had it in my mind that all women are entitled to one moment of dignity in their lives and I thought it fitting that it should accompany the coming of new life.

So I served Patsy, who didn't have the strength to turn me away. She asked only whether her midwife knew she was in labor, and she relaxed each time I said yes. Gratefully I watched the power stealing over her. I called the midwife. She had just arrived, just tucked back a strand of Patsy's hair and praised her, when a doctor barged into the room, grabbed Patsy's chart, noted that her temperature was 99.6, one degree above normal, and announced her unfit for a midwifery delivery. Without apology or further explanation, he evicted both the midwife and me. When he did that, I believe he destroyed one of the very few opportunities that ghetto child would ever have to experience human dignity and mutual trust.

I stood, appalled into silence.

"It wouldn't be done that way in England," the midwife spat. "There, we rule the unit."

Her remark led me to the mistaken assumption that midwife rule-of-a-unit would mean more respectful births. As a result, I made up my mind to study midwifery in Great Britain. While I flew over the Atlantic, miserable about leaving home, trying to staunch the flow of tears, I emboldened myself with all the stories my father had told me about being a World War II bomber pilot. I must have been thinking that my mission had moral equivalency.

Well, it wasn't war, but that gloomy brick hospital, erected high on a Glasgow hill, resembled a military headquarters. On the outside, its walls were smoked with a century of soot. On the inside were endless shadowy corridors, along which we student midwives passed, our rank marked by ominous white caps that had wings as proud as the eagle's. But if we sailed above the patients, the institution spread, in parallel structure, over us. Quartered in a "block," watched by a "home warden," we slept in metal beds and ate at designated hours. We were to starch our uniforms to boardlike stiffness and keep our civvies in a metal locker.

Clustered around the base of the hill, living in moldy tenements, was, in the bland language of the institution, our "patient population." Living in the aftermath of Glasgow's heady days of industrialization, they breathed ashy air, made do without vegetables and milk, married to get away from home, dressed their children in drab clothes, passed evenings in smoke-glutted pubs, and endured, as I have written before, the cutting of their episiotomy stitches by impatient husbands.

The Sisters, as the nurses were called, as if compensating for the infestation in the city, were compulsive about sterile regimes. It seemed like a counteroffensive to the rankness below, a boot-camp shock treatment, as if the women, like raw recruits or prisoners of war, had to be rearranged, rewritten, made to meet a higher standard. We denuded them of their identity. We shaved them, scrubbed them, and dressed them in identical uniforms. Demonstrating mastery over their bodies, we flooded their rectums with green soapy water and made them have bowel movements.

"We all had been or had fancied ourselves to be somebody," Victor Frankl wrote about his experiences in a World War II concentration camp, but by the time the Nazis had stripped them down, "the prisoners saw themselves completely dependent on the moods of the guards." So it was with our women. By the time we had accomplished our purification rituals, a midwife could waltz into a room, freely ram her fingers into a woman's vagina, and dictate: "You'll be at this all night." And the women, broken and obedient, would be.

It was the longest year and a half of my life. My energy was drained by the insatiable bleakness around me. And like the keening of winds on the moors, the memory of the voices of the senior sisters still chills me: "Today we have an arrested labor in bed twelve, a diabetic in bed seventeen, a low-lying placenta in the adjacent bed, and three sections scheduled." I see the high-ceilinged delivery rooms, the plastic hoses dripping Pitocin, the stretchers screeching down the hallways, the babies separated from their mothers by a block of corridors. I remember how routinely women's worth was desecrated.

To this day, I hate many of those midwives,[3] as I hadn't been able to hate indifferent doctors. The midwives were women, and they shouldn't have been bent on humiliating other women. But they did. I tell myself to be forgiving: In that hospital so many of the midwives were themselves victims of a punishing and humiliating system. I want to forgive, but it's hard. For I watched them transfer their abuse to the women they cared for, and I knew we would never be done with it.

Less often, but sometimes, I hated the birthing women for being powerless. Sometimes I wanted to shake them, yell at them, insist that they stand up for themselves. But then I'd feel the pull of an undertow; I'd feel them wanting us to abuse them: I'd feel them pleading for the repetition of the pattern in their lives. My fury would die. I'd realize that I'd been angry with them because they didn't want my respect.

For, unlike me, the women in that blighted city had not learned as they grew up that being female was honorable. A woman in Glasgow was born a burden, an economic encumbrance in an industrial town that had outlived its usefulness. She was not respected for her own being. Even less was she valued for the capacity she had to bear a child, a child who perpetuated misery, a child who would be one more soul who was hungry, cold, and out of work. It was then that I began to believe that if a woman knows that she and her children are not valued, she will beg to be effaced. She will want her power denied. She will deny it herself.

At the same time, I also understood that those of us who care for her will be sorely tempted to respond accordingly. When we see a woman's lack of confidence, we tell her that we will take care of her. In the doing, we can make her feel more helpless. Then we see her fear, and it may occur to us to think of her as a coward. Suspecting we have a coward on our hands, we decide we'd better do her birth for her. As we do, we feel contempt.

We are human and we may collude. When we do, we compound

a woman's feelings of worthlessness and we ensure the perpetuation of the illusion that women cannot give birth with power.

Some Conclusions

We wanted to make birth safer and less painful. In the doing, however, we disconnected birth from its source. As in so many of our dealings with the natural world, we did not understand the complexities. We didn't realize, as the physicists did not realize until their work on the atom, as farmers are only beginning to understand today, as all of us, becoming more cognizant of the fact that we can destroy the environment that supports us, that science is a complex and reciprocal affair. We cannot pull out the few mechanisms we can identify and manipulate them without reference to the whole.

We separated a few working parts of the woman from the whole of birth, we separated the birth from the whole of the women, and we separated the woman and her family from the whole of re-creation. We severed her connection with the eternal and made her more mortal, more discountable than she has ever been. We made it impossible for her to speak of powers that precede, accompany, and surpass her. We denied her material for the stories she might tell her daughters about the origination of life. We made her mythless.

We think of how lifelessness, paradoxically lively, reproduces itself; of Don Bergstrom, in his seventies, whose first child was born in 1938. His wife's doctor, Bergstrom said, sounding as so many of us do when we want to assure that we have done our very best, was "the cream of the crop" and so he deferred to him when his wife was in the hospital. Deference required that he be separated from his wife; deference required that he be excluded from the labor ward; deference required that he have no place in the proceedings. The institution, that is, claimed the right to prevent Don from witnessing the birth of his child. A man may see death—indeed institutions insisted, through World War II, that Don make his ties with death—but when it came to birth, he was unwelcome.

The doctor suggested that Bergstrom "go out and get drunk like men usually do," which is interesting, too, because drunkenness numbs life. But there was nothing else offered to Bergstrom to do while he was being barred from creation. His experience, not coincidentally, resembled that of his wife, who could do nothing either, once she was etherized. In the absence of her liveliness, the doctor used metal objects, forceps, to do what nature, numbed, could no longer accomplish.

"I'll not forget when they finally let me in," Bergstrom said fifty years later. "I looked at my wife and she looked like she was dead. She had no color. It was just like she was dead.

"You can't imagine the feeling that that arouses," he said, dead sober. " 'I killed my wife.' " It crossed his mind that he should never have sex again.

He said it was a crazy thought, but one wonders. If sex is about life, creation, and the joining of human spirits, and if it turns out, as it did in that 1938 hospital birth, to issue in deadliness, then one is not crazy to think of renouncing it. One must suspect, for a moment, that the universe seeks only destruction and that we are its sexually driven pawns. The one thing a human might do is to refuse.

So we did much more than diminish women when we conducted births in antiseptic fashion. We abolished a creative force from all our lives. We took away our opportunity to witness. Not being able to feel it engulfing us, male and female, mastering us, caretaker and mother, asserting eternality, family following family, we made ourselves smaller, more finite, and less hopeful. Encountering life, we turned our backs and studied death.

PART III

PERPETUATING THE LOSS

Introduction

WHEN SHE is not in Austria or Australia or farther-strewn places on the globe, Eva Reich, doctor, birth reformer, and daughter of Wilhelm Reich, the philosopher, lives in an old, small, white clapboard farmhouse near a small village in Maine. The contents of her tiny front parlor, in which she grew up, appear to have been jettisoned from an attic: There's a dusty piano, made inaccessible by stacks of books on the floor, a dull chrome examining stool (upon which she sits), an oak table stacked with shifting papers, a straight-backed chair, an odd-pillowed window seat, and a wood stove. A well-intended hostess, Reich puts water on for tea, then becomes so absorbed in spilling out the findings of her lifetime quest for the easy birth ("the one hour labor *is* possible in the [primip]") that she talks through five minutes of its persistent whistling.

Her head is as full as the parlor and her thoughts are as peripatetic as her life: Maybe, she says—speaking of rumor she heard that women on Cat Cay Island in the Bahamas had babies in an hour—maybe it's because they're eating a lot of seafood, they're outdoors a lot ("Do you know the work of John Ott? That light helps make a female pelvis?"), they have vegetables and they walk a lot. Maybe, she says, labor is stalled when fear is in the room ("The fear of the attendant obviously transits to the patient"). Maybe, she says, modern women have trouble with birth because they sit straight and rigid in office chairs too much and their pelves are too tight. (She stands and sensuously rotates her sixty-plus-year-old hips for us, illustrating the appropriate movements for birth). And maybe, she says, introducing a subject that would consume the next hour of her discourse, maybe it's because most birthing women experienced trauma when they were born, the trauma was encoded in their brain, and when they go into labor themselves, the old codes direct it.

While we see that the tea gets served and the woodstove gets fed, she talks breathlessly about the history of rebirthing, critiquing the movements and countermovements within it as she goes. Fascinating us with extreme possibilities, she describes the experiences of people she has guided through rebirth. Some say they "love being hugged [by the birth canal] when they slide out"; others obviously struggle for breath, wince, and draw back when they reexperience the feeling of forceps clamped on their foreheads.

Witholding judgment on the efficacy of rebirthing claims, we say, "Supposing the message *is* encoded, supposing that one can retrieve the experience, what's this got to do with good birth?" "Ah, yes," she says, scrambling for a scrap of paper, "a good question." She draws a short vertical line with a pen she's taken out of our hand. It is, she says, a representation of a shoot coming out of the ground, the beginning of a tree. We nod. She draws an arrow pointing toward the bottom of the line → If you put force on the sprouting trunk, that is, if you bend it, pinch it, or twist it, the tree grows off center for its entire life.

We wait. She waits. She watches us intently, requiring us to understand that rebirthing is reborning, that is, a recentering to one's original self. Apparently satisfied with our faces, she says, "The baby's experiences, because they are first, they are the most important . . . perinatal events affect the baby's whole life."

We think as we drive away, burdened with the names of hundreds of people from all over the globe who are making on- and off-beat experimentations in birth and rebirth, that Reich may overestimate the significance of one life experience, i.e., birth, in the formation of the individual; or, to put it another way, she may underestimate the recuperative, health-seeking propensity of life. But like her father, who is highly regarded for contributions to philosophy and tolerated therefore, for some of his untraditional experiments, Eva Reich has made, among her admittedly broad speculations, a valuable, analogic contribution to our thought. If humans are organic, i.e., growing things, then if you prune them, bend their shoots, hit them with a lightning bolt, their growth is diverted.

The analogy, in any case, fit well with the history of birth, which is human and which has, therefore, organic qualities. For when we put women in the hospital, denuded and restrained them, we inflicted a wound upon birth. Having done that, not understanding what we had done, we nevertheless began to compensate for it. As a tree grows thick and curly around a severed branch, our birth practices have become gnarly. We compensated for the wound. We concentrated on pathology. We became, indeed we continue to become, more adept in managing the problems of birth, but our growth is convoluted and tightly grained.

The past, in other words, is still with us. Despite birthing rooms, despite "family-centered care," despite Lamaze and the craze in the seventies for natural birth, the way we perceive and manage birth is inspired by the wound, by fear of pain, and by their compensatory partners, the needs to protect and control. The past, in other words, not only perpetuates itself, but proliferates in the culture and institutions of the present. It persists in the practices of doctors and midwives, in the institutions of birth, in the perceptions of people who are becoming parents today, and even among those who are birth reformers.

All of which would be too dismal to think about were we not organic. Because, notwithstanding Eva Reich, the organisms of nature, including humans and history, do heal themselves. The hard gnarled ring eventually closes around a wound and the trunk above it may rise straight, even-grained, and true, and we are verging on a healthy, straight growth pattern of birth. We already have methods and institutions—albeit few and scattered—for assisting modern women who do not live in farmhouses and do not have sisters, aunts, and cousins in the immediate neighborhood to give birth, in fact, as Amish women do: with physical freedom, psychological security, tolerable pain, unencumbered health, and with family.

Birth, we will see, is nearly solved. Thanks to midwives, doctors, psychologists, experimental thinkers like Eva Reich, and, last but not least, the traditional lives of women, we have most of the tools, science, and wisdom we need. We even have proofs.

We are timid about trusting them, not because they are not sensible, but because we are habituated to the wound. We are still, in the analogic sense, compensating for it. To correct, to get to the straight growth, we need only to understand why and how we—doctors, midwives, childbirth educators, and people having babies—are still bound to wounded birth.

The Obstetrician's Culture

CURIOUSLY, IT may be the physician and not the woman who is more tightly held by the wound. Still expected to be the scientist-hero rescuing laboring women-in-distress, he's given all the responsibility for the outcome of birth when, in reality, he has only some of the control. When one thinks of all the factors that contribute to birth outcome—genetics, nutrition, exercise, family, psychological preparedness, birth climate, and so on—the burden accepted by obstetricians is preposterous. It implies that they should be able to reverse all that has compromised a woman's birth beforehand.

It's an idea that's propagated from within and without the profession. For example, in a 1988 article in *American Baby* magazine, David Danforth, M.D., editor of an obstetrics text, was asked to guess what will be in store for women and babies by the year 2000. Danforth says: "The big change for the future in obstetrics is the absolute control of labor"; that is, "medicine will be able to direct the dilation of the cervix and orchestrate uterine activity." The advantage: "preterm labor could be prevented."[1]

As desirable as such intervention is for preterm labor, Danforth's prophecy tends to perpetuate a troublesome illusion. It promises the consumer that medicine will be able to do all. The consumer believes it and sheds responsibility onto the doctor, who must then be a god. In headlining "absolute control," Danforth makes out-of-hospital factors invisible and in-hospital factors visible. Instead of acknowledging a hand-in-hand effort, one that recognizes that women, society, and medicine working together can best reduce preterm labor, for example, Danforth may lead us to believe that in the future, we—the nonobstetrical lot of us—won't need to do anything about preterm labor ourselves. The doctors will take care of it for us.

The 1988 National Commission to Prevent Infant Mortality reminds us, as have countless other studies and commissions, that medical solutions to problems of risk are inadequate. "Sophisticated technologies and great expense can save babies born at risk," they say, but other factors outside of physicians' and technologists' purview create the risks: "The lack of access to health care, the inability to pay for health care, poor nutrition, unsanitary living conditions, and unhealthy habits such as smoking, drinking, and drug use all threaten unborn children."[2]

Is the problem of preterm babies Danforth's? Or is it ours? Are obstetricians responsible for seeing that maternal and child health is improved, or is it their job to stand at the end of society's production line and repair what society and nature have distorted? One would like to think that Danforth meant: When society fails, when we have done everything humanly possible to prevent preterm labor, then obstetrics will be able to take absolute control. And he probably did mean that. But one suspects that Danforth didn't come right out and say that because he and his fellow obstetricians haven't got much confidence in in society to improve prenatal care. So much of what a physician learns about birth militates against it.

The Education of an Obstetrician

Consider the 1985 edition of *Williams Obstetrics,* [3] the most widely used textbook in the United States today. Eleven hundred slick pages long, it is a text in process. It slips back and forth between reformist and conservative principles. A lengthy endorsement of vaginal birth after cesarean section (VBAC), for example, stands against atavistic ones like "a cleansing enema is generally given to minimize subsequent contamination by feces." Reading it, one is bandied from decade to decade, lurched from a mechanical to an organic view of birth.

Of the eleven hundred pages, twenty are devoted to the "Conduct of Normal Labor and Delivery." Starting off softly, the student obstetrician is advised that "from the first prenatal visit a conscious effort should be made on the part of all persons involved in the care of the mother and her unborn child to make the point that labor and delivery are normal physiologic processes." And, to be sure, the self-care routines that contribute to normalcy are well outlined. In an earlier chapter we read a discussion of exercise, diet, employment (debatable in the last trimester), travel, education (a woman should call her doctor about "persistent vomiting, vaginal bleeding, swelling of face and hands"), bathing, bowel habits (low-tech prunes for constipation), drugs ("with rare exceptions, any drug that exerts a systemic effect in the mother will cross the placenta to reach the embryo and fetus").

Also introduced are all the tests that can be ordered to ascertain whether problems exist: amniocentesis, amnioscopy, fetoscopy, ultrasonography, amniography, fetography, stress and nonstress tests, and so on. The clinical pros and cons of each intervention are evaluated; the psychological ones are not. But leafing through the first part of the book, one feels a reasonable balance between an interest in normalcy and safeguarding against risk. The text seems to meet its own obstetrical criteria: "It is essential for the physician who assumes responsibility for prenatal care to be very familiar with changes in normalities as well as abnormalities imposed by pregnancy."

The balance shifts when the laboring woman arrives at the hospital door. Admitted, she is to be put on a bedpan with her legs widely separated in order to "facilitate scrubbing her introitus [the opening of the birth canal] and the anal regions" with particular attention being given to the "vulvar folds." This is followed by "shaving or clipping . . . on the lower half of the vulva and the anal region." Then the enema, blood samples, blood pressure, pulse, respiratory rates. With these traditional rites completed, limited normalcy resumes. A woman may sit in a chair or assume whatever position is comfortable for her on the bed. As meager as the freedom of movement seems to a midwife—she would say, "Do whatever you feel like doing"—the offer is surprising. What about the omnipresent fetal monitor? Its output may be distorted if she's lounging in a chair.

Williams deals with this. "Haverkamp and co-workers (1976–1979) have demonstrated that an equally satisfactory outcome for the fetus can be achieved without continuous electronic monitoring of the fetal heart rate, continuous intrauterine pressure recording and fetal scale measurement, *if the mother and fetus are closely attended by appropriately trained labor room personnel* [emphasis in text]. Given a choice, most women would probably prefer the reassurance of the nearly continuous presence of the obstetrician or a compassionate well-trained obstetric associate to that of a metal cabinet and its wires and tubes that invade her and her fetus."

The obstetrical student might find this paragraph ambiguous. It clearly says that humans, i.e., "labor room personnel," can do just as good a job as fetal monitors, but it's wishy-washy in terms of how human care affects the women. It appears that human care is something "nice"—perhaps like painted and curtained laboring rooms—but not always possible and certainly not necessary for good outcome.

Probing further, however, one picks up the scent of a revolutionary concept. Is *Williams* suggesting that the fetal monitor, which many couples think of as being the highest possible protection they can buy, is no better than an experienced, "compassionate" labor room nurse? Or, worse, could it be that the fetal monitor is something less? That it does not represent the best care, as so many think, but pared down, institutionally efficient, assembly-line treatment?

That's disruptive enough. And it doesn't even address recent evidence that overreliance on fetal monitors might, in fact, be destructive to the process of birth. Dr. Edward H. Hon, the inventor of the fetal monitor, speaking at a 1987 conference on "Crisis in Obstetrics: The Management of Obstetrics" stated "firmly that 'Not all patients should be electronically monitored,'" and more strongly, "most women in labor may be much better off at home than in the hospital with the electronic fetal monitor." Dr. Joseph Seitchik (University of Texas, San Antonio) gave related testimony. "Evidence is accumulating to indicate that environments that provide attentive bedside physician and nurse services to patients with functional dystocia [prolonged labor] have a higher incidence of patients who deliver vaginally."[4]

Given the evolutionary nature of *Williams Obstetrics,* it seems quite possible that its next edition will incorporate recent studies that reveal the importance of environment and companionship during labor. If it does, however, we will be in the thick of things. Such a concept upsets the obstetrical system. Does it make sense for the obstetrician to be a "nearly continuous presence" during labor and delivery? Is he making best use of his education when he sits by a woman's bedside for hours? Is it economical for a person equipped to manage the most delicately balanced cases of life and death, to "avoid time pressures and be there [for the normal birth]," as one obstetrician recommended? Isn't it far more logical to conclude, as did another obstetrician, "I don't have the time or the inclination to do that. It's not my thing."[5]

But while we have been digressing on the merits of the fetal monitor, our *Williams* patient has been laboring. "If the bladder is readily palpated [felt] above the symphisis [the pubic bone]," we read, "the woman should be encouraged to void [urinate]." This too raises questions. Does it mean that a woman loses her ability to know when to go the bathroom when she goes into labor? Or is it that she should be going more frequently? If the latter, why don't they tell her to go every hour or so? Surely, if labor is a normal physiological process, she can do that. Furthermore, wouldn't the palpation and the motherly encouraging "to void" have the effect of wresting control from the woman and infantilizing her?

One searches for other explanations. Apparently the laboring woman is not quite in control of her body. So we might assume that she is strapped to the fetal monitor after all and needs some help getting undone and up. Or else—of course: anesthetics. The student remembers reading that one cannot expect a woman to abide her pain. One should support her wish to labor without anesthetic, but one shouldn't be surprised, and certainly not punitive, if the woman doesn't make it. "Although psychoprophylaxis [mind over pain] will not be completely successful in many women, it should be available for those who desire it and are willing to make the effort. At the same time, the woman who attempts psychoprophylaxis but finds the discomforts of labor to be too great should not be denied relief provided by appropriate analgesics. It is not unusual for Lamaze prepared women in the United States to receive some narcotic analgesia or even epidural anesthesia during labor."

And that explains the curiosity of the bladder, whose transmission lines would be dulled along with all other lower-torso sensations by these measures.

When the time for delivery arrives in *Williams,* normalcy rather drastically retreats. "The most widely used and often the most satisfactory [delivery position] is the dorsal lithotomy position [she's on her back] on a delivery table with leg supports [i.e. stirrups]. This tradition, which *Williams* has not yet reevaluated even in the face of the abundant evidence that the dorsal lithotomy position is usually counterproductive for the birthing woman, is reinforced by photographs of the vagina and vulva framed by drape.

Following those is a closeup of scissors cutting the perineum, which, the text warns the student, is getting thin; it is "almost at the point of rupture with each contraction"—recalling Joseph DeLee. "Failure to perform episiotomy invites perineal lacerations and some degree of permanent relaxation of the pelvic floor with its possible sequalae of cystocele, rectocele and uterine prolapse." Five line drawings of episiotomy repair conclude the chapter on normal labor and delivery.

Residency

While normalcy and nonnormalcy run neck and neck in the medical school text, interventionism wins out during an obstetrician's training. It's an environment in which natural birth—as one renegade obstetrician put it—is considered "an extravagant act." Amy Roselle,[6] a resident obstetrician in a large county hospital in the Southwest, concurs. In her residency experience, she says, natural birth is an exception and when it does occur, it's discounted. She remembers that one of her colleagues assisted a couple through the natural process; he floated out of the birth room, transported: It was "wonderful."

But out in the hallway among his peers long enough to realign himself with local reality, he began explaining away the grace of the birth. The couple was "nice." They were intelligent. They were middle-class. They were well prepared. In his opinion, it seemed only nice, middle-class people can succeed. Amy, who has had experience with all manner of women giving birth perfectly well at home, noted the absurdity: "It makes you realize how abnormal it [the expectation of the resident] gets to be."

Generally speaking, obstetricians-in-training do not have the opportunity to familiarize themselves with the processes of normal birth. Even at enlightened institutions like Pennsylvania Hospital, a state-of-the-art tertiary care center that has a midwife-run Birthing Suite, residents do not train in normal birth. Valerie Jorgensen, one of the very few attending obstetricians who takes advantage of the suite (doctors may practice there if they conduct their deliveries as midwives would), says, "Residents . . . never see this birthing center, never see the birthing room, never do a delivery there. . . . They very seldom see or are involved in normal birth. . . . They're not even getting a taste of this."

Jorgensen, who is in her forties, laughingly refers to herself as a geriatric in obstetrics because of the generational chasm between her training and that of residents today. "When I went through my residence program . . . we had no such thing as a monitor, we had a lot of bed deliveries because we had only two or three delivery rooms . . . and people who didn't need the delivery room delivered in beds. I think we got a sense of comfort that the woman would not cave in if we had unassisted vaginal delivery."

It was partly in response to the absence of a normal climate that the Birthing Suite was opened. Bruce W. Herdman, Ph.D., a hospital vice-president instrumental in the development of the suite, said that the doctors and administration felt their institution was excellent in specialty care. And, indeed, the cover of the department's glossy 1984–1986 Triennial Report advertises their expertise with a full-color photograph featuring a surgical tray in the foreground and seven masked/hooded/gowned figures surrounding a mound of green drapes beyond. One of the figures holds a successfully ex-tracted neonate.

The hospital was not, on the other hand, offering much to the couple who wanted a techless birth. "There is a risk that even the husband is going to get an ultrasound if he gets up on the [traditional labor and delivery] floor," Herdman quipped. Yet that is what the residents see day after day, that is where they learn their routines, that is how they develop their understanding of what birth is like. There is no plan to have them rotate through the Birthing Suite.

Pennsylvania Hospital is not an isolated case. David Gandel is a Rochester, New York, obstetrician whose philosophy of birth has swung from the "poetic" to the "alarmist" and back to somewhere in between. (His anxiety shot from the poetic pole to the interven-tionist on the first day of residency. "There was chaos. Two patients with abruptions. Both bleeding profusely. Another delivering quin-tuplets. Stat c-section and all the babies died.") Perhaps because he has settled on a balance between the two attitudes, Gandel has been active in developing strategies for normalizing Strong Memorial Hospital's labor and delivery floors. At this time though, he said, "Residencies are problem-oriented. . . . Obstetricians are trained to jump in and do things abnormally."

These individual reports match up with what Diana Scully ob-served during fieldwork in two urban teaching hospitals. In her 1980 book, *Men Who Control Women's Health: The Miseducation of Obstetrician-Gynecologists,* Scully writes that "training developed in residents a sense of identity closely linked to the role of surgeon and that taught them to achieve their primary work satisfaction from the act of operating."[7] The pressure to be surgically skillful is so strong that "within medicine, obstetrician-gynecologists are said to have a 'cure complex.' That is, residents derived satisfaction from surgical intervention and were frustrated by less aggressive medical treatment."[8] And "the training program . . . emphasized the type of skills needed to handle pathological conditions and acute situations."[9]

In an aside, Scully wondered if the tendency to overmanage arises not from educational necessity but from the personalities of people who enter obstetrics. "There is evidence to suggest that power and control are important to the obstetrician-gynecologist. In fact, several physicians suggested that rather than interview them, I should administer personality tests to them; they believed that they as a group would score relatively high on manipulative or Machiavellian items."[10]

Others have made similar observations: Lynn Payer in *Medicine and Culture* reports: "The British medical student Dr. Eleanor Moskovic, who spent some time at Massachusetts General Hospital, noted, 'There seemed to be an overwhelming number of so-called 'type A' [compulsive] personalities around.'"[11] Payer, who gives other examples of American medicine's aggressiveness (our comparatively high rate of hysterectomies, for example), suggests that doctors may be no more and no less aggressive than Americans at large.

In addition to these softer, psychosocial explanations for the manipulative nature of obstetrics, there are also some hard, practical ones, which put stronger pressure on the resident every year. In Jorgensen's "geriatric" age, before the explosion of high technology in medicine, the resident had relatively limited surgical and medical expertise to acquire; today, however, she or he must become proficient in an ever-updated phalanx of exotic testing and machinery. "They are so involved with trying to weed their way through this tremendous array of sophisticated equipment," Jorgensen says, "that they think that pregnancy means high blood pressure, diabetes, or something else drastically wrong."

We hear echoes of her conclusion seven hundred miles away at Dartmouth Hitchcock Hospital in Hanover, New Hampshire. George Little, a pediatrician and chairman of the hospital's department of maternal and child health, says something similar: "That there has been a contamination, if you will, of the birthing experience by technology and knowledge and attitudes is a valid argument." Intriguingly, his view merges with that of external critics of the system. Diony Young, director at large for the International Childbirth Education Association (ICEA), observes that "lack of training and experience in uncomplicated obstetrics together with heavy reliance on sophisticated equipment, such as electronic fetal monitors, prepare many young physicians poorly to handle uncomplicated labor and birth."

While residents do not have an opportunity to become familiar with the normal birth process, neither do they have much opportunity to acquire caring or interpersonal skills. To the contrary, the system discourages their development. Scully: "Like other physicians, residents . . . believed their interaction with patients had to be impersonal and objective and socialization was incomplete until the resident was able to accomplish with ease the transition from person to problem."[12]

One need only join rounds to see the attitude being inculcated. The white-coated bevy of residents, anxious and competitive, gather round the attending physician and they move, a peripatetic tribunal, from bed-end to bed-end. The women, vulnerable and small, tucked in bed, look up at the surrounding experts who discuss their cases. Occasional questions are thrown at the woman and her answers are translated into data for the clinical discussion going on among senior and junior physicians, none of whom derail themselves from their left brain to bend over and touch a woman's arm, let alone catch a breath of her emotional state. There isn't time, for one thing; but more than that, one feels the presence of a powerful taboo. The resident is obliged to produce information and clinical analysis on the spot; the patient, at least during rounds, must remain in the clinical position, as if between laboratory slides.

Jorgensen, who believes that "ninety-nine percent of medicine is translating to a person what is going on and interpreting for them," remarks that physicians aren't known for their communication skills. Not only do they fail to explain, she says, they fail to listen. "It's a very difficult thing to get them to do. Even to get them to listen to one another."

"We were not listening to what the mother had to say," one midwestern hospital–trained maternity attendant remarked. "We would ask, 'When did you feel the baby moving?' If they said it was at a time when you didn't expect it to be, you discounted it and wrote down what you thought it should be."

Paltry communication skills may go with the territory. According to *American Health,* patient-doctor communication has broken down. Citing a report co-authored by Frederick Platt, MD, for *The Annals of Internal Medicine,* they say that doctors may learn a high-control style. " 'As physicians go through more specialized training, they seem to learn a bizarre approach to patient interaction,' says Dr. Platt. 'They don't know when to shut up and listen. They ask so many questions, patients can't get a word in edgewise.' "[13]

Jorgensen has an idea that the noncommunication factor may be due to the fact that medicine has traditionally been male-segregated and suggests that many men have had less opportunity than women to develop listening skills. George Little takes a more philosophic view of the origins of the problem. "It is very difficult to be at the cutting edge of creation of new knowledge and the rigid application . . . of the scientific method," he says, "and simultaneously be at the same cutting edge in the art of . . . working with people in a personal sense." He believes that Dartmouth Hitchcock is one of the few institutions in the country where there is a concerted effort to attend to both aspects of health care.

Jorgensen and Little may be speaking to the same point. In both their remarks upthrust the familiar divisions between the male and female traditions, between the rational and emotional, between mind and body, between body and soul. In medicine, particularly, it seems damned hard to get the two sides to mate.

Amy Roselle, the resident we mentioned, gravely misses the soul side of practice. Attracted to medicine because she wanted to care for the sick, to heal and to comfort, Roselle is finding that residency shows little respect for such gifts. It is not only that the institution most rewards surgical and medical expertise, that it depersonalizes in the name of efficiency, but that the long stretches of being on call—thirty-six to forty-eight hours—leach her emotional resources.

"I am more cynical, less happy. I tend to be pretty outgoing, smart alecky in what I think is a pleasant way, but—maybe it's sleep deprivation—but I get tearful, short, then feel guilty and then I get upset with a patient." For Roselle, the impersonality of the program is so destructive that she has considered leaving. She fears having her softer side destroyed. "I think I might have to put my real self into a cocoon for the four years of residency. If I don't . . . the emotional side of me will be swallowed up."

What Roselle speaks of as a personal conflict is being posed by some today as a legitimate medical issue. Some scientists are investigating the degree to which emotional and psychological factors affect physiological ones. We see the possibilities being explored in popular works like *Love, Medicine and Miracles* (1986), Dr. Bernie Seigel's best-selling book, which draws on studies implying a substantive communication between mind and body. He preaches that what people believe and how they feel about themselves have a profound effect on their resistance to disease and, in fact, on their ability to cure themselves of disease. The physician, Seigel argues, can augment the healing process by listening to his patients and teaching them to listen to themselves. The physician's touch, hug, "being there" enables well-being.

The same issue is also explored in the more sophisticated *The Healer Within,* which deals with the relationship between the immune system and one's emotional state. Early in the book the authors, Steven Locke, MD and Douglas Colligan, establish that medicine today is losing or has lost its human touch.

> Physicians themselves are beginning to see that technology has diluted some of medicine's more humanistic elements, simple parts of the medical ritual, like touch, that have genuine therapeutic benefit. This new consciousness can be found with increasing regularity in the pages of their leading journals, such as the *Journal of the American Medical Association* and the *New England Journal of Medicine.* The message is that our phenomenal progress in medical technology has had a certain cost: "Recently I visited a ten bed intensive care cardiac unit," mused one physician. "The Faustian soul of modern technology had provided that most touching was mechanical, through electrodes, wires, tubes, scopes, and the like. Medical professionals were

rarely in contact with patients." Another doctor commented: "The specialist-physician is metamorphosing into a technocrat and businessman. The physician retreats behind the machine and becomes an extension of the machine."[14]

The question is: Is the machinery, as it replaces the human, in the best interests of health, specifically with regard to the immune system? The authors of *The Healer Within* suggest that while most people intuitively know that those who are touched and cared for are healthier than those who are isolated, explanation of and proof for the correlation has, so far, escaped us. " 'Knowing' that one's state of mind influences one's body does not prove that it does," they write. The trouble is, gathering scientifically admissible evidence requires researchers to sail over the edge of the scientific flat map; it calls for the mingling of the less containable science of psychology with the more easily encased laboratory studies of immunology. " 'Most immunologists,' " said one of their number, " 'are naturally uneasy and usually plead not be be bothered with such things.' "[15]

While the book demonstrates the difficulties of experiment design and the vagaries of results, the evidence has a cumulative impact. Somehow, in a complex way, people who are cared for, who care for themselves, and who care for others seem to do better in immunological matters. Therefore, "there is real medical power in the healing touch of the caring physicians."[16]

A point we infer from reading Scully, that may not be completely lost on those residents she was following around. While they are pushed in the direction of the mechanistic model during training, most of them said they intended to add a caring factor to their practices. They expected to call out their hibernating humanity and remember the injunction in *Williams Obstetrics* that they should make a concerted effort to communicate to the woman that pregnancy and birth are normal processes.

Practice

Alas, the workaday world of today's obstetrician does not invite the breaking of habits acquired in medical school, neither with regard to caring nor with regard to a normal perception of birth. Caring requires attention, attention requires time, and time is money. If our Amy Roselle, wet-winged from her cocoon, wants to go into practice she must come up with about $37,000 (1987) for one year's medical malpractice insurance fees before hanging out her shingle. The tab is likely to be on top of outstanding medical school loans. This puts her under considerable pressure to get a high return from a day's work. George Little, the Dartmouth-Hitchcock chief, describes what happens: "We're always talking about efficiency and we're always talking about how many patients per hour we're seeing. What is the productivity of the individual physician?"

One might plead with Roselle to choose the noble road and commit herself to living modestly, paying back her loans slowly, and "being there" for her patients. But that's tough. "There are insurance companies, third-party providers constantly, increasingly, questioning how much one should be paid for a particular procedure or unit of time. . . . In other words . . . if a couple is in for a prenatal visit, you are allowed ten minutes for that prenatal visit," Little says. "Suppose that you have plenty of office space and that the computer works fine, the telephone works fine, and you get into the office [on time]. It's still a situation where Blue Cross/Blue Shield or Kaiser or somebody says they're allowed . . . say ten minutes. . . . There's another appointment at 3:10. . . . And the things we've talked about today [caring for the whole woman], some of the needs we've discussed, don't come that easily."

It makes more sense for Roselle not to go it alone. Better to join a group practice or get work in a Health Maintenance Organization (HMO). But then what happens? Responsibility for the individual patient is distributed among several OBs, some nurses and nurse-practitioners. There Roselle signs up a patient, plans to see her for her prenatal care—excepting deliveries, vacations, and emergencies—but she is obliged to make it clear to the pregnant woman that the odds of the two of them meeting on the labor and delivery floor are one in four or five. That's up to the fates, expressing themselves through the on-call schedule of the obstetrical group.

Under these circumstances, Roselle is compelled to become more technically oriented. Even if she wants to be generous with her time and her human nature, in the back of her professional mind is the very real need to prepare a record that will serve any of her colleagues (or a resident). Her precognitive impressions, her intuitive judgments, her interpersonal hospitalities are not so fit for charting. What is fit are test results and hard data; what might help are a couple of extra ultrasounds. Thus relationship is thwarted; thus pregnancy is technologized.

Generic Malpractice

Although the medical malpractice epidemic is among the most commonly cited causes of overmedicalized birth, we have put off discussing it. We have delayed not because we doubt that it is a major contributing factor, but because we wanted to establish that it is not the only factor. Solving the medical malpractice crisis will not "solve" birth care because the crisis is as much a symptom of our problem as it is a cause.

Having said that, it is important to acknowledge the truly poisonous effect of malpractice litigation on the relationship between caregiver and client. It has become a perverting agent. Meant to protect individuals against a minority of incompetent or malevolent practitioners, the law has been applied against a majority. By 1987, 71 percent of American obstetricians had been sued at least once—a rate suggesting that obstetricians can be trusted only in the exception. This makes for an unhealthy climate in birthcare.

Obstetricians admit to feeling paranoid. Some sorrowfully say that they have come to see clients not as human, not even as machines, but as potential litigants, snakes in the grass. Given that climate, their exchanges with patients become guarded; instead of thinking about the patient's needs, they think about how their advice will sound to a jury's ears. To protect themselves, they warn excessively against the hazards of birth. "Don't be alarmed if the caregiver spends a lot of time going over the risks involved in pregnancy, labor and delivery," a popular magazine advises the pregnant woman. "In the past, neither doctors nor patient cared to dwell on such dangers, but many of today's practitioners insist that patients understand them."[17]

Roselle says, "Medicine is so . . . political and legally oriented and compulsive. . . . I see my peers are concerned about what is going to pass in court: If I do this, am I liable? The documentation, what is said, what is decided, what is explained. It's not a standard of care; it's what we do to cover our asses."

Litigant pressure forces the practitioner to build a patient chart that will stand up in court. The more interventive, the better. "When pressed as to whether aggressive treatment is really better, American doctors often answer that they must treat aggressively or get sued for malpractice. There is some evidence in support of this: "American . . . law tends to require that everything possible be done for the patient, and doctors certainly believe that juries will be kinder on their sins of commission than on their sins of omission."[18]

The fetal monitor, which Jorgensen calls the "gold standard" of obstetric care, "turned it [medical practice] around." She says it changed physicians' methods of managing birth. It also solved some of the courtroom's evidentiary problems. Obstetricians, lawyers, and judges have always had to live with confusing differences in professional opinion, with judgment calls, with the varying standards of practice from medical community to medical community, and they still do. But readings from the fetal monitor seemed to make things simpler. They have the distinct advantage of being tangible proof. The "strip," the piece of paper that scrolls out of the fetal monitor, has evidentiary hardness. It is replicable, quantifiable, and comparable to other strips. Thus one may take a strip, and read it (rather than talking to a woman or touching her body) not for her sake, but for the court's.

The overuse of the fetal monitor is only one example of how medical malpractice claims have influenced birth care. Thinking about charges that could be brought against them, practitioners tend to overtest. They must systematically prove the absence of potential complications, even the most remote. They test for diabetes, they order numerous ultrasounds, assume that a patient should have an amniocentesis, and may urge other, more exotic tests just to make sure they've covered themselves. The more nervous the patient—read, the more likely to sue—the more screening. The more screening, the more anxiety. The more anxiety, the more indications of physiological stress, the more stress, the more intervention, etc.

When the woman arrives in the hospital, they "take that strip," or leave her on the monitor; they insert an IV, and, in a bizarre twist, they may perform major surgery, the cesarean section, with its attendant risks, in order to prove in court that they followed the safest course of action.

Thus legal pressures transform relatively normal patients into abnormal ones. "Physicians," said Bruce Herdman, the vice-president at Pennsylvania Hospital, "drop patients on our [high risk obstetrical specialists] all the time because they don't want to take the responsibility for this patient or that." Thus, in parts of Florida, that high-malpractice-insurance state, the cesarean rate has risen to 40 percent.

Everyone seems to agree that there is a correlation between cesarean rates and litigation rates and many believe that if we can just unsnarl the serpentine relationships between insurers, physicians, and the public, the problem will go away. A lot of energy goes into the effort. Doctors plead with parents to give up the naturally absurd notion that every child will be a perfect child. Birth reformers nag at physicians for performing surgery unnecessarily and causing emotional and physical damage to their patients. The American College of Obstetricians and Gynecologists goes against prevailing practice when they recommend vaginal birth after cesarean section. On a television talk show, Mortimer Rosen, MD, chairman of the department of obstetrics and gynecology at Columbia University in New York City, advised women to seek a second opinion when their doctors recommend cesarean. Insurers, who often require second opinions in all other incidences of major surgery, are following suit. In the meantime, they travel the country and teach physicians how to weed the legally risky patients from their clientele.

But one wonders if we aren't so absorbed in the particulars of the medical malpractice crisis that we fail to consider its root causes.

Maybe the fracas is not about malpractice in the specific meaning of the word but, given the number of suits, about malpractice in the generic sense. The courtroom language may veil a much more serious discontent. If we have sued 71 percent of our birth caretakers, we may be saying that we sense something fundamentally wrong with the way we are conducting births in this country. Maybe we "just know" that birth care has become distorted. We can't say why because we don't know the language, because the explanations are not available to us. We can't argue with the experts because they are occupied by arguing among themselves. We can't offer alternatives because we don't know what they are. We feel angry. There is nothing else to do, so we sue.

And maybe the obstetrician is also trapped. It can be argued that we have set the physician up. We absolve individuals of responsibility for birth and teach them that doctors can fix anything. As a society, we fail to provide prenatal care for many women and then we criticize doctors because they cannot correct for the effects of our stinginess. We ask doctors to learn all the latest resurrective techniques and then we charge them with thinking like machinists. We leave them ignorant of the marvelous vagaries of natural birth but insist that they believe pregnancy is a normal life event. We ask them to undertake work for which they are not well prepared—i.e., normal labor and delivery—and then wonder why they make the task complicated enough to suit their skills. We ask them to respect women, but we require that they work in a setting that routinely infantilizes women. We want them to be sensitive to the multiple factors at play in a birth, but we cleave to the illusion of absolute control. We tell them to "be there" for a woman, and then we stopwatch their time. We ask them to be wise in the art of medicine, to bring all their experience, intuition, and compassion into their decision-making, and then we evaluate them on the basis of data produced by machines.

We may be bringing suit against doctors for reasons we don't understand. We may be attacking them not for their individual professional failures but for the failure of a national fantasy, the one that said medicine was to be certifiably, verifiably, uniformly, mechanistically miraculous. Maybe we are angry because nature turned out to be more complicated, more difficult, more multifaceted than we had hoped it would be back there in the early years of the century. Maybe we all made a mistake. Maybe we missed the mark. And wouldn't we be wiser to consider the possibility that 71 percent of individual American obstetricians are not in the wrong, but that there is something wrong in our way of thinking about birth.

The Midwife's Culture

I F ONE of the disadvantages of late-twentieth-century American life is that we have painted ourselves into an obstetrical corner, one of our advantages is that we don't have to invent our way out. We can dip into the experience of a multitude of other cultures and use their experiences to advise our own. We can search obstetrical science and practice in other countries; we can draw on the knowledge of professional and lay midwives in our own cultures and others; and we can always—a fascinating excursion—learn from the experience of a worldful of women who have assisted one another at birth.

From a practical point of view, however, we are fortunate in that we don't have to travel far nor do much translating from culture to culture. At hand are the experiences of American nurse-midwives. They draw on the same knowledge base as do obstetricians. They have legitimacy (the American College of Obstetricians and

Gynecologists recognized them in 1982 as members of the health-care team) and they serve American women.[1] They relate, in other words, to the same broad culture as American physicians do.

On the other hand, they represent a strand in that culture different from that of doctors. Almost all of them are women and they also draw, as we will see, from women's culture in their profession. Because of this, they practice a distinct type of birthcare. If nothing else, nurse-midwives give us another perspective on American birth practice. By examining their culture, attitudes, and professional habits, we gain added perspective on problems and solutions in the birthplace.

With Woman

The most obvious difference between American obstetricians and American midwives is that the former tend to manipulate nature more aggressively than the latter. Knowing what we do of the history of midwifery, we can see why. Practicing among pots and pans as they did for so long, midwives didn't have the luxury—or the temptation, for that matter—of becoming overly sophisticated. While they took from medicine what they needed, they also relied on domestic tools at hand.

Midwives practiced for years in woman's traditional environment and, as a result, they inherited many of the attitudes and practices of the mother of the house. Instead of perceiving their clients as medical cases, midwives have been more inclined to see woman in the way that mothers have seen their family members.

Mothers have traditionally nurtured the health of their family members in what some today call a holistic fashion. They have always been responsible for feeding, clothing, educating, and playing with their families; for monitoring happiness and sadness; for planning outings, holidays, and family gatherings; and for bringing beauty into the home—the geranium on the windowsill. In the twentieth century, of course, mothers' responsibilities have become more complex. In addition to managing the external factors of the family's life, today's mothers are concerning themselves with inner states. The nineteenth-century child who didn't eat, for example, was put to bed, ignored, whopped, or bribed. Today women are expected to deal more subtly. When today's child refuses to eat, mothers are to consider emotional well-being. Has something happened? Are there inappropriate tensions at the dinnertable? Is some school failure manifesting itself gastrointestinally? We asked a young, well-read homemaker what her intellectual life consisted of: She said, "I try to understand why my son behaves the way he does and what it tells me about his needs."

The homemaker's tradition is holistic when she uses emotional and psychological therapies in combination with medical ones when she cares for her family. If, when children are ill, she takes them to the doctor, gives them necessary medication, she is using scientific sources for healing knowledge. When she fixes them their special favorite foods, sings to them, changes their pillows, lets them rest on the couch, rubs their backs, airs out their rooms, and talks to them, she is using domestic sources of healing knowledge. From pragmatic experience, she knows that stories read out loud soothe and heal. She may not be able to explain why she fusses so—although love has something to do with it—nor why attention seems to heal, but she's likely to buy medicine *and* Crayolas when she sees a long illness setting in.

The midwife also combines the scientific and the domestic. In addition to her medical knowledge, she thinks about the room in which a woman gives birth—its wallpaper and curtains; she wants to know what a woman feels like eating; she asks a woman questions about how she feels about babies; she asks after family members; she tells birth stories; she soothes; she calms; she reassures by her very presence.

Calling attention to these hominesses, however, may imply that midwives are not as sophisticated as they claim to be. It might be more appropriate to dignify motherhood/midwifery traditions by connecting them with that trend identified by Locke and Colligan, authors of *The Healer Within,* the ones who suggest that body and mind do interact in ways we can't quite yet explain. Better to pull out Norman Cousins's testament to the value of laughter in healing or cite Leonard Sagan's book, *The Health of Nations* (1987), which provides some epidemiological evidence that progress in our public health statistics may have as much to do with *hope* as it has to do with improvements in the public health system. For tone, we can cite Thomas Mann's *Magic Mountain,* which slips feverishly from body to soul. For international chic, we can let drop the French medical concept of *le terrain,* the idea that the body is a kind of soil that must be nourished by life or even left to lie fallow—as in going to a spa.

The nondomestic, nonintellectual world, too, has begun to sponsor holistic health thinking. Consider the behavior of big business. Corporations build gymnasiums so their employees can sweat off stress. We see on television that Steve Allen's son goes on corporate lecture tours, giving therapeutic laughter sessions; someone else demonstrates relaxation methods and another T'ai Chi. If a bank teller is shot in the course of a robbery, squads of social workers charge in afterward, ready to guide employees healthfully through their trauma "work." Presumably these investments pay off in reduced sick leave.

We look at random in the culture at large and see how holistic we are becoming. Our interior decorators design for peace and health, putting plants and aquariums in waiting rooms. Architects of skyscrapers, considering "human factors," make microparks just outside revolving doors. Lawyers send clients to therapists. Therapists send lonely people to the pet store to buy themselves a companion. Neonatologists discover that premature infants who are touched and held thrive better than those left isolated in their perfectly clean plastic boxes.

While we might say that we have a growing holistic climate in our institutions, no one really understands why or how emotional and environmental factors influence physical well-being. Some things we can prove—the restaurant decorator probably has numbers that "prove" that bright red prompts rapid turnover, as in McDonald's— but so much remains, in the strict scientific sense, unproved. As compared to the medical model, it all appears to be a trifle kitsch. Obviously this presents problems for the midwife, whose practice would be better legitimized if its holistic aspects were more amenable to weighing and measuring.

The Education of the Midwife

The 1980 edition of Helen Varney's *Nurse-Midwifery,* the most widely used text for student midwives in this country, is conservative. The human touches are in there, but the text clearly favors the medical model. Thus, the model birth is in a hospital delivery room—complete with its table, lithotomy position (modified), draping, gowning, scrubbing, and instrument trays. *Nurse-Midwifery* does not exclude the possibility of other settings—labor or birthing rooms, for example—and it says that the principles used for delivery room births can be "extrapolated for preparations for delivery in other settings"—but we read about the delivery room.

In the second edition of the text, however, published in 1987, we see some reclamation of the domestic tradition. Varney's done more research, spent time with practitioners in other settings. She describes birth center and home births, she analyzes the effect of physical environments, she dispenses with hospital-specific requirements and adds those that are necessary to the out-of-hospital setting. In other words, she makes the extrapolation.

But before we follow this homey path out—and in 1987 Varney took a leap—we should give some attention to the medicine of midwifery. This is not only in deference to the medical competence of midwives, but also because it allows us to see how midwives think and, for that matter, haven't yet thought.

Nurse-Midwifery[2] is medically conscientious. We find drawings borrowed from Moore's *The Developing Human: Clinically Oriented Embryology,* and *Williams Obstetrics.* We can study E. A. Friedman's famous labor curve, "Primigravid labor: A graphicostatistical analysis, reproduced from Obstet. Gynecol 6:569, 1955." We read that fertilization is the "fusing of the female and male pronucleus from the ovum and sperm respectively" and that subsequently "the fusion of pronucleus of each gamete restores the diploid number of chromosomes, which is subsequently reflected through mitotic cellular division in every cell . . . except those which later undergo gametogenesis." In other words, it presumes specialized knowledge.

It explains how to screen for antepartal complications like incompetent cervix, hyaditiform mole, ectopic pregnancy, hyperemesis gravidarium; it tells about infections with exotic names: toxoplasmosis, cytomegalovirus, and condylomata lata, which we must not confuse with condylomata acuminata and so on. The lay reader is reassured to see some familiar diseases discussed—things like herpes and gonorrhea; it reassures us that we are reading about the parts of the body we were originally interested in.

We flip through an exhaustive list of items to be considered in physical examinations and antepartal exams and are regularly reminded that a prime purpose of such exams is "to evaluate the woman for normality and to screen her for medical and/or obstetric disease or abnormality." We are told time and again that a major responsibility of the midwife is to spot indicators of problems that the physician must diagnose; her alliance with him or her is a commandment of midwifery.

We can study structural variations in the pelvis, learn about the muscular action of the uterus, turn the book upside down and sideways and, looking at pictures, try to visualize the positions the baby's head might take vis-a-vis certain bony protuberances. We are taken slow step by slow step through the physiological processes of normal labor and delivery. Ultimately we read how to manage complications like placenta praevia, cord prolapse, and postpartum hemorrhage until the doctor arrives or until the operating room is prepared.

We notice parallels in style between *Williams* and Varney. Both books present all sides of debates on state-of-the-art issues. In some instances, we find the same debates—both books evaluate the risks and benefits of amniocentesis, for example. But Varney differs from *Williams* in taking up some humbler issues. Enemas, for example, are assumed in *Williams,* presumably because they have long been thought to clear out space-taking debris and thus make more room for the baby's head in the pelvis, and also because they make it unlikely that a woman's body will, during expulsion of her baby, contaminate the sterile field.

Yes, but . . . we read in Varney. Yes, but if the woman doesn't "want" an enema she may retain it, thus defeating both purposes. Yes, but if she is deep into labor, she may expel the baby with the enema. Yes, but the enema may provoke cord prolapse, or—if the membranes are already ruptured—intrauterine infection. "It becomes evident," the text concludes, "that routine enemas for all women do not constitute good management."

On the other hand, it continues, enemas can stimulate labor and if the labor needs stimulating, if the head is well engaged, if the membranes are not ruptured, if the enema is the least intrusive stimulation, then it may be appropriate therapy. In other words, the enema should not be considered as a routine measure, but as an optional low-tech intervention.

For the most part, however, Varney and *Williams* are in congruence regarding strictly medical matters. Clearly the midwives have adopted that part of obstetrical science that pertains to normal birth and made it essential to their education.

Human Skills

We said that doctors weren't encouraged to be emotionally and psychologically sensitive during training. Midwives, by contrast, are required to do so. Ploddingly, painstakingly, the midwifery text teaches its students to listen. A midwife is supposed to be "tactful and respectful of a woman's right to privacy." She must maintain eye contact: "Don't always be reading from the history form, writing responses, charting." She should credit a woman's perception of her body: What is the "woman's evaluation of her own health status?" She is expected to develop empathic skills. "If a woman is talking about a past difficult time in her life . . . sympathetic understanding is appropriate."

"Listen to the woman . . ."

"Listen to the woman . . ."

"Listen to the woman . . ."

For the midwife, the "normal data base of pregnancy" is not just physical, but emotional and psychological as well. Pregnancy is "a time of transition between what life was like without this child and what it will be like with this child." The pregnant woman has "labile" feelings. She is "vulnerable. She fears death for herself and her baby. She is frightened of the unknown because her body seems out of her control and her life is in the process of being changed irreversibly."

We learn that each trimester brings emotional change: ambivalence, anxiety, and concern with weight in the first; maternal identity-seeking and emotional storehousing in the second; watchful waiting, birth anxieties, and nesting in the third. Midwives are urged to practice "honest sharing" with the couple in these matters.

Consideration and openness carry through into the physical exam. The midwife should warm her own hands under a hot-water faucet or underneath an examining light before she touches. She should talk about what she is doing as she goes. "Share your findings with the woman. If she is anxious about something that you find normal, immediately tell her so." There is a law implied in *Nurse-Midwifery* that is missing in *Obstetrics:* "Remember, it is the woman's body." So, the text explains, there will be women who will not want to have a pelvic examination. "Such women will be both mentally and physically hurt if an attempted examination is forced upon them" and therefore one should not force it upon them. Better to talk, to listen and to wait.

It's important to note the text doesn't work out the physiological value of respecting women and their bodies. It does not mention the possibility of a relationship between victimization, loss of control, and poor progress in labor. It does not suggest that the woman who is not hurt during a prenatal exam is less likely to be fearful of birth—and thus "better" at it. It doesn't examine the interaction of fear and labor hormones.

Which is to say that *Nurse-Midwifery* reflects that baffling aspect of "state-of-the-art" health care in the eighties: It recognizes that emotional and psychological factors are significant in birth but it can't describe the circuits connecting them to physical ones. Varney simply asserts that psychological matters are part of pregnancy and birth and that they are, therefore, a part of good care. As a practical matter, this may take Varney's students beyond Williams's, but it does little to demonstrate why the emphasis is correct. The case seems to depend on a common appreciation of the value of compassion.

It may be indicative of trends in health care thinking that Varney's humanistic bent grew more robust during the eighties. Consider her discussion of grief in the 1980 edition. She says grief is current throughout all pregnancy and birth: There is the grieving of the newly pregnant woman who has lost her old way of life; the grieving of the newly delivered woman who has lost her intimate physical relationship with her baby; and there can be the grieving of the mother and father who have lost a newborn. She presents the stages of the grief process and suggests how the midwife can support the woman or family as they pass through them.

By the 1987 edition, however, she shows a stronger conviction about the importance of emotional factors in childbirth. Not only does she continue to emphasize their play in pregnancy, but she even breaks from the relative safety of the psychological sciences. The text punctures the clinical capsule. It quotes the poetry of a grieving mother, Lois Lake Church:

Not Mine

Powdery scent, apricot-soft skin
of someone else's infant . . .
Mine only, these big-belly memories,
mine the not-to-be-fulfilled dreams.

So there it is. Brave, tradition-breaking testament to the mother's voice and to the poetry of birth and death. Language of the home and heart. Bold assertion of a holistic philosophy, and we think for one inspired moment that we are on the verge of a breakthrough— that Varney is going to button body and soul together for us.

She doesn't. She can't.

Thinking Like a Midwife

Having said that Varney does not prove a connection between sensitive care and good health does not mean that midwifery is not well founded. If nothing else, midwives can prove the efficacy of their techniques by their outstanding statistics. They do have unequivocal evidence that their way of practicing does "just" work. They even have some physiological proof organized. Furthermore, midwives have an intellectual discipline and critical method for evaluating procedures. Very much simplified, it involves weighing three factors: What is healthiest? What is most comfortable? What is the least interventive?

To see how these three factors work in a midwife's analytic process, let's start with a common procedure—the shave around the opening to the vagina, or perineal shave, and see how a midwife evaluates it. Reminding ourselves that none of the three factors can be evaluated without considering the reciprocal effect on the others, we'll consider comfort first: Does the woman like to be shaved? Or, ridiculously, does it make her feel good? Not likely, the midwife would say—having perhaps experienced the itchy aftermath of the shaving procedure herself. So that's something against doing it. (For emphasis, we note that Varney does *not* mention that a woman's labor might retreat when her private parts are approached by a razor blade.)

The question of whether the perineal shave promotes health, however, requires a more complicated answer. If an episiotomy is planned, then a shave could make sense: A micro-shave right around the opening to the vagina might prevent errant hairs from infecting the stitching. But then, being suspicious of all intervention, a midwife might ask whether it's necessary to do an episiotomy in the first place. If it's not done, one can eliminate (a) the risk of the contaminating hair and (b) the uncomfortable (inhibiting) shave—not to mention postbirth swelling, prolonged irritation, etc.

But we can't question the episiotomy until we know whether it can be avoided. We have to believe that it's possible for the midwife to produce this clinical feat—the uncut opening of the vagina, or intact perineum. Because the midwife will insist that the intact perineum is only partially attributable to her hand skills, we are required to look more closely at her management of human and physical factors in childbirth.

The midwife teaches the pregnant woman about exercise during pregnancy, although not the aerobic kind, which is good for her heart and lungs, and not by toughening the muscles on the pelvic floor—making them hard, the way one might wish one's stomach muscles to be. For birth, flexible muscles are best, ones that have been repeatedly stretched and relaxed. The idea is to make the pelvis and all its attached muscles movable and spreadable. So, for example, one English birth educator and yoga teacher recommends that women get down on their hands and knees every day and and "make slow sexy circles with your hips. . . . Now rock your hips backwards and forwards."[3] Belly dancing and squatting have the same salubrious effects.

Flexibility complements birth. The muscles and bones are looser. They are well oiled. They are conditioned to give. They are prepared to respond to the changing shape and placement of the baby as he travels through the pelvis.

Which is what one has to imagine next. When a woman goes into labor, her baby's head is usually sunk down against the cervix (the opening of the uterus), which, conditioned by hormones, has softened. If one touches the unpregnant cervix, it's like touching one's nose; if one touches the "ripe" cervix, it's like touching one's lips.

Contractions, which start in the upper uterus, wave downward. The process is like forcing frosting through one of those fabric cake-decorating cones—squeeze at the top end and a coil of frosting comes out at the pointy end. The pressure continues in its wavelike fashion until the baby's head, in search of the path of least resistance, presses against the softened cervix, which effaces and becomes fully dilated.

As soon as the head gets into the birth canal, things change. Up to this point, the laboring woman has been concerned with making herself as comfortable as possible while her body worked for her: lying, sitting, pacing, standing in a shower, or wallowing in a bath. When the baby's head enters the birth canal, however, she—the part of her that can "do something"—becomes active. She generally feels a compelling need to push.

As we imagine the baby moving into and through the birth canal, we can understand the value of natural labor. If the mother's pushing is not retarded, as it can be by an epidural, the baby travels fast enough—and the caregiver has less reason to cut a swath to hasten his exit. If the contractions are not overaccelerated, as they can be by Pitocin, the baby won't come driving down like a boxer's punch, which tears the perineum.

In natural labor, the baby's head spreads the opening gradually, in keeping with the mother's own musculature and tissue. Moving along at a rhythm and pace defined by the mother's anatomy and physiology, the baby's head serves as a well-timed prod. It burrows along, budging the birth canal open before it as it goes and ultimately stretching the perineum, whose tight aperture gradually gives way, opens up, and lets a little light fall on the baby's head. It's quite an amazing thing to see, this yielding. One never imagines its being possible and yet, there it is. The perineum, which turns out to be soft and expandable, like a doeskin pouch, swells and ripens before your very eyes, very fruitlike. There are pictures of it in *Nurse-Midwifery*.

Now we are at the point at which we can understand the origin of the midwife's rule that "there is no one way to give birth." The mother who is free to move will experiment until she finds a position that feels best. She rotates, she thrusts, she writhes (those belly-dancer moves) to find the most expedient method of getting it over with. As she does, she generally accommodates the baby's progress. She makes room. These squatting or semisquatting positions midwives talk about so much are not mandated but have been discovered by women giving birth. One might get rational about it and speak of the advantages of working with gravity, of keeping weight off blood vessels, but during the expulsion phase of labor the woman is directed by her body. The attraction to squatting is just that, an attraction—one that happens to abet the expanding pelvis and perineum.

Mind you, the midwife has not "done" anything yet, that is, not unless you count the education during pregnancy and the support and monitoring during labor, but with the head on the perineum the midwife can act. Her goal is to help the head get past the perineum without tearing. She is working with a bulging head, fierce contractions, and a woman who is not sensible in the usual sense of the word.

From the first time that midwife and client meet, they are creating the *terrain,* or ground, for this moment. All the conversations, the questions and answers, the touch of the midwife's fingers on a woman's belly, the comfort measures, the respect shown for feeling and belief, all the months of exchange, the little bits of life passing back and forth, the minute human events that seem not worth reporting have been preparation. Having been woven into the relationship between midwife and mother, they finally produce trust. They bind voice to ear and touch to touch.

Which is necessary because the time between pushing contractions is like the lolling of the sea between waves and the laboring woman seems to drift down into a half-light below, where the midwife must reach her. Her words are simple; her voice is firm, direct, sometimes oracular: "I want you to release your breath through the next contraction. Phuh. Phuh. Phuh." The woman, her eyes drifting and her head lapped against the pillow, may nod slightly, wasting no strength, before the contraction closes in, clasping the baby's head tight to the perineum. "Phuh. Phuh. Phuh."

Once again the sea lolls.

The woman grunts once.

"Again," the midwife says.

Twice.

The head, lightly propelled, slips out through the perineal ring.

The Practice of Midwives

Building the kind of trust which complements birth is time-consuming and time, we remember, is what physicians have trouble getting. Midwives fare better in the delivery system in this respect. For one thing, they are less burdened with overhead. They are not as heavily endebted for their education. It doesn't cost them as much to set up an independent practice or for a hospital to bring them on staff. Because they are less reliant on technology, their routine expenses are lower; because they give some nursing care themselves, they require less support staff. Because they are not (yet) often sued, their malpractice insurance is relatively modest, averaging $4000 a year. Having made education, counseling, and support a formal element of care, they are generally permitted by insurers and hospital bosses to linger with clients. Thus midwives can and do spend more time with women—spending twenty to twenty-five minutes with patients as compared to doctors' five to ten.

The one time problem midwives do share with physicians is that of getting to births. For the childbirth practitioner, doctor or midwife, it's virtually impossible to be at every prenatal exam and at each birth *while* looking after enough patients to make a practice pay *while* getting enough sleep *while* setting aside enough time to be with their families *while* attending their own health and sanity. Thus, midwives in hospitals, birth centers, and in independent practice, like doctors, do work shifts and do cover for one another.

Certainly the shuffling of patients has some of the same disadvantages for the midwife as for the physician—i.e., it discourages the development of intuitive exchanges and the building of trust, but the midwife may at least include emotional/psychological factors in her history of her client. Thus, sitting in a staff meeting of eight midwives at a large hospital, one not only hears summaries of the patients' physical condition, but also, "Her boyfriend has decided to marry/ not marry her; her husband will come to the birth/go to California; she does/doesn't like to be touched; she is excited/terrified/disinterested in the prospect of birth." In other words, the emphasis on human factors is considered relevant information among midwives and is, therefore, charted and tracked.

In general, then, midwives may suffer less from institutional and economic pressures than physicians. They are allowed to spend more time with a patient and they have the latitude to be more sensitive and intuitive. On the other hand, they encounter obstacles specific to their profession: Their freedom to practice at their best is hampered by the state of obstetrical art, by biases within the medical community, and, in a terribly complex way, by the clients themselves.

Some of the disagreements between obstetrical and midwifery practice are subtle, difficult, and worthy of debate. How a practitioner presents the risk factors inherent in tests is a good example. The alphafeto protein (AFP) test, for example, is meant to show the absence or presence of a certain protein in the mother's blood. If the protein shows, then the baby could have a spinal defect—e.g., spina bifida. In the spirit of informed choice, therefore, all mothers are to be advised of the availability of the test, a requirement that many doctors fulfill by saying, "It's time for your AFP." Midwives are more inclined to present a more complete picture—one that includes information about the limitations of the tests and the ethical and emotional issues they raise.

Five out of a hundred women having the AFP will be told that the test reads positive. Unfortunately, however, the AFP is only a first screening, and those five women must then undergo further tests in order to determine whether their child has a disability: These include amniocentesis (which has a 3 in 1,000 chance of causing a miscarriage)[4] or ultrasound (the long-term risks of which are unknown).[5] Only after these tests are completed is it possible to determine which one or two of the five women are carrying a potentially disabled child.

Midwives certainly do not argue that these tests are inappropriate. What concerns them is the neglect of emotional factors in the presentation of the choices a woman or couple must make. Since the tests don't tell how serious a problem might be—they can range from the mendable (after birth) to the severely disabling—a more complete rendering of the decision includes: Is the woman/couple willing to abort a child who may have a minor disability? If they do, and find out that the fetus was not severely afflicted, how will each of them live with the long-term consequences of taking a life? How will it affect the partners' perception of themselves as parents and their parenting of other children?

Then, too, midwives would argue, such elaborate, serial testing may well undermine a woman's confidence in her body. Having a test to see *if* everything is okay certainly suggests that it may not be. If the message is repeated by a series of tests, the woman learns to distrust her body—a feeling likely to discourage her from giving herself over to her body during labor.

Testing may also restrain her emotional attachment to her child. In *Tentative Pregnancy,* Barbara Katz Rothman shows that some women don't feel the child moving until after an amniocentesis confirms that the baby is all right.[6] In other words, the woman might cancel out her baby's communication—i.e., "He moved"—until an external apparatus advises her that it is safe (the child is healthy) to fall into relationship with her baby. While no one suggests that this is disastrous for the parent-child relationship, there is loss implied. That subtle, almost smokey talk between a mother and her unborn child can be mysterious, lyric, and delicately sweet, and one can't help but think it destructive to hamper it unnecessarily.

Midwives do not suggest that there are easy solutions to the problems raised by testing, but they do find themselves in conflict with physicians who define the problem clinically, who toss off the procedures as if they had no human ramifications. Midwives argue that the pregnant woman will be a mother for the rest of her life. The feelings she has about her child during her pregnancy, the decisions she makes about her or him, will accompany her to the end. Midwives wish physicians would consider the emotional consequences of their recommendations and decisions.

Because they involve the relationship between mind and body, these disagreements between doctors and midwives about testing are legitimate and difficult. They need time to be considered and developed. Far less tolerable are unadulterated power plays between the two camps. Many hospitals, for example, essentially delicense out-of-hospital midwife practitioners at the door. So a midwife from a nearby birth center may accompany her patient to admissions and then lose all professional say in the care of the patient. She may remain as a support person, but her professional opinion, and with it, the woman's birth choices, are rendered null and void.

One home-birth nurse-midwife tells of a woman in early labor whose baby was discovered to be in an odd position—instead of being aimed downward, its head was directed toward the pelvic wing. Often such a baby will squirm around during labor and ultimately find the path of least resistance, but it's not the sort of thing one leaves to chance. The midwife explained to her very committed-to-home-birth couple that they would have to go the hospital and that she, conscious of their sensitivities, would be pleased to accompany them. All the way to the hospital, the husband kept asking, "Is this really necessary?"

"*This,*" the veteran midwife pronounced, using her life-and-death voice, "is necessary."

Once at the hospital, the midwife, couple, and physician reached a gentleman's agreement that the woman would continue to labor and that a cesarean would be performed only when it was clear that the baby wasn't going to redirect itself. Knowing that the woman was still in the earlier stage of labor, the midwife left to get something to eat. When she returned a cesarean had been done. "Why?" the midwife asked. "It was easy," the physician responded. "Everything was set up for cesarean in the delivery room." The gentleman's agreement among doctor, midwife, and couple was ignored; the clients paid with bodies and pocketbooks. The midwife, their advocate, had no authority within the hospital walls.

Midwives working in a large Pennsylvania hospital found they were unable to prevent the anesthesiology department from setting policy that would allow anesthesiologists to approach every woman in labor—even during transition—and describe to her the much blessed relief she would feel with an epidural. Although this is sabotage, midwives were not permitted to interrupt the sell to inform the woman about the disadvantages of the epidural, which the anesthetists glossed over.

An experienced midwife in another large urban hospital sometimes assisted residents at deliveries. Being new at the process, the residents often encountered situations that were frightening to them but familiar to the midwife, who provided some input. Hearing about the midwife-to-resident teaching, one of the senior physicians criticized his younger colleagues: "Don't let that midwife push you around. Why are you doing what the midwife is telling you to do? That's not an appropriate way of being a physician."

Laurie Friedman, a Yale-trained midwife now practicing in greater Boston, suggests that the problem with certain physicians is that they "are coming from a perspective that believes that there isn't any such thing as a normal birth." Like Valerie Jorgensen, the OB at Pennsylvania Hospital, she makes a distinction between younger doctors and older ones. "I think a lot of midwives find very satisfying working relationships with physicians who were trained before there were fetal monitors and before there were fetal scalp samplings and before there were ultrasounds. Because they have the skills . . . relying on your hands . . . to decide what position the baby is in or how strong the contractions are. All those kind of things are things that physicians had before the development of all this technology. The residents . . . don't have those skills because they rely on ultrasound and fetal monitors to give them that information."

Thus the conflict with the midwife's philosophy, which relies on the primacy of a woman's experience. They put their energy into "patient education . . . empowerment and facilitating [the woman's] being able to make choices about things." For the high-tech practitioner, these tend to be no-account factors in birth. They can't be machine measured. Therefore, they are invisible; they are not considered factors in birth, they are not data. They don't exist.

And so we are faced again with the issue of who and what controls birth: Should it be the technologically trained physician, utterly reliant on technological data, who assumes that he must be in control of the birth, or should it be the woman, equipped with knowledge of her body and her feelings. Friedman argues that total physician control undercuts birth: "When you take away a woman's power, when you violate her ability to participate, when you treat her like a patient in the hospital, you mess up the way the birth is going to go and you make it impossible for her to have a low-intervention, good-outcome birth." In other words, the physician's overemphasis on technical data, his command posture, distorts the birth process.

Friedman is not optimistic about the possibility of an easy reconciliation between high-tech obstetricians and midwives. In her view, the possibility of their finding common ground retreats faster than it advances. Starting with conception, she says, with the idea of in-vitro fertilization, women may think more and more of reproduction as a laboratory phenomenon and less as a human one. Our engagement with these medical miracles—which she does not condemn—reinforces the public's perception of birth as a process that ought to be technologically controlled, a view in direct conflict with that of a midwife. The two "perceptions" she concludes, "are not intertwinable."

With these forces in play, it should not be surprising to find that the other major challenge in a midwife's practice is women. "But how do you get them to take responsibility for their births?" student midwives ask experienced ones. "How can we get women to participate in their births?" members of the audience asked Michel Odent.

Suzanne, a midwife at Dartmouth-Hitchcock Hospital, had had some home-birth experience in Connecticut. Women would come to her and say, "I don't want to end up with forceps." It was as if the midwife, like the doctor, was supposed to be able to produce a birth. The nonforceps delivery, Suzanne said, "was something we were supposed to deliver." Similarly, Charlotte Houde, the director of the nurse-midwifery program at Hitchcock, talks about a woman who wanted a binding contract that she would not have a cesarean. She insisted upon the agreement throughout her pregnancy—which was complicated—up to and including the last minute, when her baby was found to be lying crosswise in her pelvis. A c-section was scheduled; the woman complained, attempting to make Charlotte responsible for everything. Although Charlotte refused—"It is time to stop having this tantrum and to start thinking about that baby"—she had to cross the woman's expectations to do so.

As that meeting in Penny's living room suggested, the problem of guiding women to birth is fraught with difficulty. Teaching women that they have say—whether they consciously exercise it or not—is a major educational undertaking, one that requires breaking the hold obstetrical medicine has on the American imagination and helping women to rediscover their natural power at birth. As much as anything, it has to do with making invisible factors visible.

A Visibility Tale

Some practitioners, doctors, and midwives, see "invisible" factors and some don't, and we would understand birthcare better if we divided them by this criterion rather than by their professional titles. It is just as the feminists have taught us: There are men who are better "mothers" than their wives and women who are better "fathers" than their husbands; there are doctors who are more "midwives" than some midwives and midwives who are more "doctors" than some doctors. There are caregivers who countenance the invisible factors that Laurie Friedman speaks of and those who don't. There are those who understand childbirth as being whole and human and those who specialize in its mechanical subparts. There are midwives who are termed minidocs because of their relative lack of interest in psychosocial aspects of childbearing and because of their readiness to "fix" a labor. The other way around, there are doctors who like to "be there," know a woman, and let her labor her own way.

Take Wendy Savage, for example. One could say that she's a midwife's obstetrician because she's invested in her clients' lives. Her practice takes shape from them. Although she works in London—which means another culture, another set of expectations about childbirth, mothering, and so on—her experience deftly illustrates the institutionalization of the conflict between the two perceptions of women at birth. At the London Hospital, Wendy found herself attacked by those who do not countenance invisible factors.

At fifty, Wendy is a senior consultant in obstetrics, which means she's an expert in the system, the person called in when the midwife, general practitioner, or resident has identified a problem beyond their area of expertise. Given the hierarchy, one might expect someone in Wendy's position to be distanced from patients, whose human qualities, if they are to be tended at all, can be delegated to those who do primary care. One of her responsibilities, indeed, is to march those residents at double-time through the wards, snapping out questions and challenging faulty obstetrical answers. Indeed, it's said that Wendy doesn't suffer fools gladly.

In spite of her position, however, Wendy's interest was in establishing a system of care that took women's rights and needs into consideration, a pursuit that did not set well with the medical hierarchy. Although she is a Fellow of the Royal College of Obstetricians and Gynaecologists—one of the highest honors the profession can bestow—she was charged with incompetence and suspended from her posts as senior lecturer and honorary consultant at the London Hospital.

One could argue that she made a likely target. Her career path, for example, was not typical. Her experience is too broad. She studied at Cambridge, took her medical training in London, did epidemiological research in Boston, practiced obstetrics in Kenya and Nigeria, set up blood banks, treated fourteen-year-old girls who had infected uteri from self-administered abortions; she practiced obstetrics and set up family planning and venereology clinics in New Zealand. By then she had four children. She returned to London.

Furthermore, her personal style is distinct. She's self-directed and very swift—we've watched her red leatherette, tie-on running shoes striding across the stage to the podium. It's not the sort of mien likely to charm gentlemanly colleagues. Wendy makes a good lightning rod: a tall, raw stick of a woman poking her bony elbows into the padded ribs of the medical establishment.

Despite the fact that she has written a book about the affair at the London Hospital, Wendy remains bewildered by it. Obviously it had to do with the rights of women giving birth; hence her title, *A Savage Enquiry: Who Controls Childbirth?* And if you ask her, "What happened at the London?" she can trace administrative and legal details with precision. She can describe the highly irregular manner in which allegations of incompetency were brought against her that were meant to separate her from her posts. She can explain that this was done in spite of the fact that her perinatal mortality statistics were as good as anyone else's in the service of the London; in spite of the fact that there had been no patient complaints; in spite of the fact that it is the tradition of physicians to defend rather than attack their own. But for this irregular woman, administrators at the London ferreted out a procedural device generally reserved for doctors who were seriously addicted to drugs or mentally disturbed and used it to accuse her of mismanagement of five obstetric cases.

After fifteen months and an estimated total of £250,000 in legal expenses, the panel of two obstetricians and a barrister who heard Wendy's case concluded that of the fifty-nine charges, "fifty-five were found," as she reports, "to be invalid or insubstantial, and in four instances there were criticisms of my management which did not amount to incompetence."[1] Thus was Wendy able to describe *what* had happened at the London.

But if, picking up the sulfury scent of witch hunt, you ask, "But why did it happen?" she appears baffled.

"My friends say, 'Why Wendy, it's because you're such a threat to them.' "

"But," Wendy says, "I can't see that I am such a threat . . . although I put things in a straightforward way. . . . But I don't know why [they did it]."

Her book puts forward two explanations. On a relatively trivial level, the affair appears to be the result of personality conflicts, in-house politics, poor communication, and administrative disarray—one of those tangled and idiotic trip wires that bureaucratic life can string across one's path. But Wendy's supporters, the women of the community she served, did not see it this way. They raised money at jumble sales for her defense fund, pushed their prams in marches protesting her suspension, appeared on television to speak on her behalf, and brought her bouquets of roses and freesias to keep her spirits up. Not middle-class women, accustomed to making organized political statements, these were the women from London's East End: poor English, Cypriots, West Indians, Somalians, Chinese, Sikhs, Vietnamese boat people, Gujeratis, and a lot of Bengalis. The majority lived below the poverty line and in council (public) housing. Neither at the time nor after her reprieve did the women see Savage's suspension as a sad administrative lapse; instead, they thought it had to do with those invisible factors we have been talking about.

I, Sheryl, took the London Underground to a stop in the Tower Hamlets section of London's East End, walked past some vacant shops, a helpless-looking newsstand, a bakery and stood, momentarily mesmerized by a display window made radiant by swaths of sari cloth. Moving on, peering through alleyways, I could see the monotonous, grassy flats upon which the brick, council-built apartments were set.

Elizabeth's flat was three flights up a blackened-brick stairwell and a few steps across a balcony, which was strung with a white rope. A few kitchen towels had been thrown over it to dry. Elizabeth, a little heavy, a little pale, very warm and pleasant, invited me in, introduced me to Peter, her husband, who was lounging underneath a spider plant that hung from a ceiling hook in the corner of the living room. Baby Matthew was asleep in his crib in the bedroom and three-year-old Heather ensconced herself on a plastic pad on the floor between Elizabeth and me, where she pounded authoritatively on purple home-made play dough. "The secret's in the amount of oil you put in it," her mother confided.

Elizabeth's childbirth experience began in a hospital antenatal clinic at the other end of Tower Hamlets. With hordes of other East End women, she went to prenatal appointments at a designated hour—block booking, it's called—sat in a room that allowed no play space for children, and waited hours for her turn to come up. "You used to see one doctor after another . . . nine times out of ten it was someone different," Elizabeth said. "At a lot of the hospitals, you would go to one department, they would treat you for this, you go to another, they would treat you for this, and so it goes on, but they don't treat you as a whole person."

In Elizabeth's case, such fragmentation may have resulted in poor pre- and postnatal medical care. Although she is an epileptic, they missed taking her blood levels during pregnancy and birth. A couple of weeks after birth she hemorrhaged, and although they did a D & C (scraped the uterus), no one told her—if, indeed, they had found out—that she was anemic.

But, intriguingly, it wasn't the medical sloppiness that infuriated her. "They don't treat you as a whole person," she charged. "You go to the gynecologist or obstetrician just to be examined for the pregnancy . . . but they don't take into consideration that it might be affecting you psychologically and that you get other ailments." She felt that her experience in childbirth qualified her to speak to this issue.

Because when she went to the hospital to give birth to Heather, she really didn't want an epidural. While she couldn't say why exactly—mainly, she didn't like the idea of having "somebody mucking about my back"—she was clear in communicating her preference to the hospital staff. "I was uncomfortable, but I said I'd rather suffer." To her dismay, the staff argued with her. "They were afraid I would have a fit [seizure]. . . . Everyone was on me to have an epidural." Although she explained to them that pain didn't trigger seizures in her, they gave her the epidural anyway, wouldn't let her push, did a "terrific episiotomy," and used forceps to deliver the baby. Elizabeth was silent for a moment, as if to make sure I had a chance to absorb what she'd said.

Canny Heather took the opportunity to pat my knee and offer me a purple pancake, which I accepted. Then I asked Elizabeth why, in her opinion, they had ignored her wishes.

"I think they're frightened," she said. "They like to be in control of the situation and if there's no need for intervention, they aren't in control. They would be in control all the way along. The fact that they're not a hundred percent in control all the time seems to frighten them."

Heather, who had waited patiently for her mother to finish, wanted to know what we thought of her creation, so we discussed the merits of the pancake, which I then had to give back. Elizabeth went on to explain what happened after her baby was born.

"I saw Heather right after she was born, but I wasn't up to it, really, at the time. They took her away and four hours later I asked to see her. They just said, 'She's all right.' "

I had my eyes fixed on the familiar tubes that Heather was rolling from her clay, but I could feel Elizabeth looking at me. "That's no answer for someone whose just gone through twenty-four hours of labor." Her voice was trembling.

"I said to them," she continued, " 'Hasn't she got dark hair?'

"They said, 'Didn't you know?'

"It was all too much trouble [for them]," she said with a faint cry, then paused. I knew my head was moving from side to side. "And then they wonder why you get depressed afterwards," she said. "Makes you sick, doesn't it?" she said. I nodded and gave in to my temptation to stroke Heather's head.

Eighteen months of postpartum depression followed the birth. In order to care for her and the baby, Elizabeth's husband lost time from work. She sought therapy. After six months of trying to figure out all the things that were "wrong," she thought that one of them might be anemia and prescribed herself some iron pills. But mostly, "I was angry with everyone, but what made me angriest was that you couldn't get back at anyone." Peter, suddenly lively, interjected that it had made him very angry as well.

In spite of the long struggle for recovery, or maybe because of it, Peter and Elizabeth decided they wanted another baby. In her pursuit of health, Elizabeth had joined the local chapter of the National Childbirth Trust, a childbirth education association, and she'd learned some things about obstetricians, midwives, and hospitals and found out that if you went to Mile End Hospital (part of the London Hospital system) where Wendy Savage practiced, a woman was treated differently.

For one thing, Wendy had set up community clinics. You could get an appointment for a specific time; you saw the same general practitioner or midwife every time. Wendy herself, senior consultant, would show up in the doctors' offices to go over a case, with the general practitioner sitting right there listening. People knew each other. The only glitch was that Wendy had been suspended from practice, so Elizabeth and Peter waited to get pregnant until she was reprieved.

Giving birth to Matthew was "wonderful. I went to the hospital [at Mile End] and everyone listened. I wrote down a birth plan. I thought hard about it. I said no epidural and the nurses never [questioned my choice]. They knew how much I was against it and they never said anything." She went on to say that midwives and residents not only listened, but they explained what was happening all the way through and they asked what you thought. If Wendy Savage's people said you needed an intervention, you knew you really needed it. "Anyone who looked after you under Wendy Savage—even if it was to wash the baby—they'd come and ask you if it was all right."

You could even see the difference between midwives who'd trained at Mile End and those that had been trained elsewhere, she said. The ones trained other places, "They're the people who are very much in charge, who don't let *you* stop and think what's best for you and for the baby. Even in the postnatal period, it was, 'You do this.' 'You do this.' 'You do this.' You get lectured to." She said their attitude didn't do much to help a woman solve the problems she was going to have to solve by herself when she went home. "It takes time to get your self-esteem and self-confidence back. It goes on a long time."

About then, baby Matthew started cooing from the bedroom, so we went to see him. His mother let me know that he was already pulling himself up by the crib bars. "Why do you think the other women in Tower Hamlets took to the streets in defense of Wendy Savage?" I asked, watching the padded nine-month-old make his stand.

"Everyone who had been treated by Wendy felt they had been treated well, with respect, by a woman, from a female point of view."[2]

And that was what we heard from others.

"She's not 'up there.' "

"She was one of us."

"She's not an honorary male."

"She knows that relational well-being is important to the birth."

"She took herself out to the community."

"She actually does see her patients. . . . I know a woman who's had three babies with [a male doctor] and has never seen him."

"She looked in on me [even though I'd been transferred to another hospital]."

"She cut a lock of hair from the head of a severely deformed stillborn child and took it to the mother."

"She takes time."

"She listens."

Leafing back through *A Savage Enquiry,* one notes that the case against Wendy had been mostly rumor and fumble until the time she objected to a reduction in the number of obstetrical beds at Mile End. She'd written out her arguments, citing the good perinatal and maternal mortality statistics at Mile End, expressing her concern about maintaining adequate services for the women of Tower Hamlets, and suggesting that the proposed changes had not been adequately costed and considered. The administration at the London subsequently described her report as "counterproductive" behavior.

Shortly thereafter the case against her hardened. Using various slippery devices, the administration dug up five of her worst cases and put them in evidence as examples of her incompetence. Wendy is the first to say that the cases were not her best and that, in fact, criticism was due, but the heat they generated was all out of proportion. As one of the witnesses put it, "I can say without hesitation that if the worst five of my own cases over the period of a year were put under a microscope, it would be possible to create a dossier similar to that of Mrs. Savage. I believe the same could be done of every consultant obstetrician that I have ever worked with."[3]

Furthermore, the focus of the charges was suspicious. They ignited on the issues of shared care—that community clinic scheme—and on the right of women to participate in birth decisions. Most dramatic was the case of a Bengali woman who wanted to try vaginal birth after cesarean section. While Savage had not been especially optimistic about the woman's likelihood of succeeding, she knew that Bengali women prized vaginal birth and so she instructed the lecturer [resident] who was to attend the birth to give the woman every chance.

Her judgment was later endorsed by one of the witnesses for the defense, a professor of obstetrics and gynecology at the University of Bristol. He testified that among Bengalis "the aversion to Caesarean section goes beyond, in one sense, what we might call reason." He said that Bengali men were known to reject their wives if they had cesarean and cited the case of one wife who had had a cesarean "for cast-iron reasons" and subsequently ended up in a mental institution. "The psychiatric opinion is that the triggering factor in a woman who was predisposed to this [mental illness] anyway was . . . her husband's response to the fact that she had had a Caesarean."[4]

Reflecting on her case later, Savage wrote, "I regret that I did not understand how opposed the lecturer was to allowing the woman to experience labor, even though I knew that the chance of her delivering vaginally was remote. Had I done so, I would have taken over the case completely." Admitting administrative error, she did not relinquish principle, "the principle that a woman should be able to have a trial of labour, even if I do not think she will succeed, as long as she and the baby are all right, is one that I stand by."[5]

Why did it happen, this nasty, protracted affair at the London? Wendy's personal nonconformity, no doubt. At the hearing, the London's administration was represented by a "phalanx of sober-suited men"; Wendy sat among "less formally dressed women." Political and administrative disagreements, no doubt. The administration at the London, it turned out, was interested in developing the institution's in vitro capabilities; Wendy's priority was basic health.

But the dispute erupted when Wendy defended services at Mile End Hospital, and it expressed itself in charges that challenged the shared-care system and the involvement of women in obstetrical decision making.

It seems to have happened because Wendy insisted on seeing women as people with lives, beliefs, and reliable birthing bodies. It seems to have happened because she insisted on taking those invisible factors into account, because when she did, the existing system exploded.

Reconciliations

T HE CONFLICT between those who acknowledge invisible factors and those who don't leaves the childbirth consumer in a kind of no-man's land. Captives of the conflict in opinions, they must flip the misnamed coins of informed choice and choose a side. They're told how lucky they are to live in a time when they are free to make the impossible choice: They can have doctors, who are the representatives of precise medical care, or midwives, who are the representatives of humane care. Few tell them that one might not need to give up the protections that medicine offers in order to have a humane birth. Fewer still launch the radical notion that the birthcare that gives weight to the human dimensions may, in fact, result in a healthier birth.

Not all childbirth professionals, however, accept the choice. A growing number prowl the no-man's land, renaming it common ground, and look for ideas that promote healthier births.

Women Obstetricians

Many women hoped that birthcare would automatically become more sensitive to women's needs when more women became obstetricians. The old male/female, master/servant paradigm would vanish. The control quotient would disappear. Women doctors would not be handicapped by the blindnesses of sex. Women doctors would have felt the slick warm flow of menstrual blood or would have accommodated cramps or morning sickness or the svelte moves of a child turning within or the feelings of insufficiency that pregnancy evokes. Women would have a natural sympathy with the power of birth and its quality of pain. Even if they had never had a child themselves, they would look upon the laboring woman with sensitivity: "She could be me."

But the reviews of women obstetricians are mixed. Fredericka Heller, a forty-year-old obstetrician who enthusiastically backs midwives, says, "If you're looking for women who are oriented toward childbirth and you think that all women coming into medicine are very female-oriented, you're wrong . . . they're following right along with what the fellows are doing."

For some feminists, this could be reaffirming. If it is true that males and females are androgynous in their learning capacity, then it follows that women attending medical school would acquire the same ideas as men students. To succeed, they would devote their college lives to competing for good grades in hard sciences, their medical school lives to attracting an offer of residency from a noted institution, and their residencies to proving mastery of technical skills. Once in the game, like Amy Roselle, they would play according to the rules.

Heller, who calls herself a female advocate, says that young women medical students are seldom aware that sexism exists, nor do they appreciate its effect on women. They "haven't been in the real world. They've been in academia—which is a fairly reasonable place to be [with regard to sexism]. They don't think prejudice exists. . . . They haven't been in the situation with lack of power, lack of knowledge."

She has. Not when she was a medical student at the University of

Pennsylvania where "I got awards for being a woman's advocate," but when she went to do her residency in the mid-eighties. There she found herself "bound and gagged for those things." It didn't help her popularity to get pregnant. "Although I was thirty-five, I was told it was inappropriate for me to have a child while in residency." Making matters worse, she expressed a desire to invite her ten-year-old son to the birth of her second child. Her colleagues were further offended.

Attended by a midwife, it "just happened" that she wasn't able to get to the birth center in time. "I had my baby in my own bedroom." And while "it was wonderful," it was not rewarded by her colleagues. Two days later, the obstetricians in her department said, " 'You're in trouble.' "

Heller sighed. "The men had gotten together a petition to have me thrown out of the hospital with the midwives [who had been practicing there] because I'd had the audacity to have an out-of-hospital birth." And although her residency was ultimately saved by the all-hospital physician staff, who overrode the decision by the obstetrics department to have her terminated, and although Heller herself has continued to be outspoken on the needs of women and the importance of "being there" at births, she does not think she is typical. She thinks that most female obstetricians—and particularly those who haven't been off the medical school preserve—are very much deterred by their male colleagues from imagining what it's like for a woman to give birth. And even if they should imagine the meaning of the experience and if they should tie it in with feminism and speak of empowering a woman at birth, they run a sizable risk of disempowering their careers.

A recent article in *The New England Journal of Medicine* supports Heller's opinion. It finds that women residents are influenced by the male standards of the institution. About "40 percent [of women residents in a study] said that their pregnancy had elicited some hostility from their program directors, and 41 percent had felt some hostility from their fellow residents."[1] Whether it was because of that hostility, or whether it was because they had internalized the standards of performance set by residency programs (we don't know), "The women in our study worked until the time of delivery in most cases, did double duty, used vacation time before and after the birth to make up for lost time, and returned to work an average of eight weeks after delivery for an average of 95 of the 168 hours per week."[2] In other words, women going through residency programs made their pregnancies and births fit into a schedule designed for the nonchildbearing sex.

Following traditional feminist lines, the report gives them credit for their performance. Yes, childbearers can perform equally as well in residency as nonchildbearers; "women have managed to meet their work responsibilities while pregnant, with a minimum effect on their programs."[3] This in spite of/because of the fact "four-fifths of the programs we surveyed had no policy on maternity leave."[4]

But then the authors (five out of the six are women) make a break from the male mimicry phase of feminism. They suggest it might not be the best thing to put childbearing last on the list of things that need to be considered in life, residency or no residency: "A physician mother should not be so pressured by rigorous career demands that she cannot spend 'needed' time with her baby."[5] More radically yet, they argue that the residency system in general, for both men and women, isn't good: "The current climate of residency is in direct conflict with the realities of a young person's life—the time needed to develop a relationship with a partner; the age limits of fertility, the time needed to carry, breastfeed and care for a baby; and the need to sleep in order to function effectively."[6] They boldly recommend an investigation into a "fundamental change in the current pressures of residency programs."

And so, like the midwives who make their case for humane care on compassionate grounds, the authors of the *Journal* article argue that you ought not to treat residents like soldiers under siege because it's inhumane. A good enough argument. One that many of us on the outside of the medical tribe can support. Why, indeed, must residency resemble a prolonged Outward Bound exercise? Yes, one wants a doctor to have learned how to work when tired and under pressure—but ninety-five-plus hours a week, month after month? The system deprives residents of life. Were it absolutely necessary—as it might be during an epidemic—then, yes; but in relatively normal circumstances, it seems suspiciously punitive. And if it's true, as many say, that those who are treated punitively, treat punitively themselves, then the patient ultimately pays.[7]

The *New England Journal* authors don't discuss the effects of such conditioning on doctors. They don't flirt with the possibility that a deprived resident might end up ignorant of life itself. They do not suggest that a person who hasn't had time for intimacy may not know its worth; they do not hint that emotionally malnourished persons may be unable to give of themselves. They don't consider the megamessage that the system communicates to its future caregivers: that wholeness is dispensable.

The postpartum efficiency standard certainly teaches that. It tells a woman resident that she doesn't need time or energy to appreciate the more complex dimensions of birth and mothering. It tells her that babies should be born without distracting the mother. It tells her that she must remain unaltered by hormonal cycles and untouched by maternal feeling; as a practical matter, she is expected to deny a major life event. The system gravely insults the mother and her child by refusing to acknowledge their existence, much less their worth.

Perri Klass, MD, wrote about her residency for *Ms.* magazine. "So we hissed sexist jokes and we applauded the use of the female pronoun," she said, striking the gongs that announced the fight for women's equality. Then, helping us understand the predicament of women in medical school, she says the women tended to merge with the status quo. "Did that mean that the women with whom I went to medical school considered themselves feminists? I can't say, but I do know this: many of us felt poised, as women entering a traditionally (and sometimes militantly) male profession, between gratitude to the women who had fought their way through before us on the one hand, and a desire to identify with our new brotherhood on the other."[8] She thought her own feminist efforts were quite modest. With a friend she ran the medical school women's association, but their activities were "far short of revolutionary."

But again, just as in that report for the *New England Journal of Medicine,* Klass gives us a whiff of something coming: "I also remember how different it felt the first time I was ever in an operating room with an all female group: the orthopedic resident, the surgical intern, the medical student (me), *and* the patient. And in fact it was nothing like the usual operating room drama; there was less yelling, more courtesy, more collegiality and less strict hierarchy. That distinction has held up in a fair number of operating rooms since then."[9]

Fredericka Heller and the *Journal* and *Ms.* articles make us remember that the feminist directive of the sixties was for women to prove that they could perform as men perform. Looking at women medical students now, we might conclude that young women did as they were told. Only now, as the first phase is completing itself, is the next one appearing. The old question was: Can women succeed in the medical field? The rising question is: Are there insights that women, specifically because of their legacy as women, can bring to our larger concern with health and healing?

We have a few indications that there might be. Heller's "female" mind advises her to "be there" for a woman, to think of birth as a natural, healthy life event, an event having to do with home, family, and wonder. The "female" mind of the *New England Journal* article also advises its authors to think of birth and mothering as an important human event, a family event, one complete with emotional and physical dimensions, not to mention time-consuming responsibilities. Perri Klass's females are more collegial, more cooperative, and calmer than their male counterparts. They work together rather than run orders down a line. The emergent theme is interdependency.

There Are Doctors and There Are Doctors

We read new studies saying that babies show personality traits at birth; we read that male babies, as little as an hour after birth, respond differently to certain stimuli than do female babies. Our surfaces, the *tabula* of our selves, may be clean when we are born, but each of our slates is unique—some are glazed, others porous; some brightly colored and vivid, others wet and thick. We call these given characteristics our gifts. How else to explain why some caregivers merge into a labor as comfortably as old sexual partners fold into one another. Penny talks of Mike Szutowitz, a family doctor she knows.

He smokes too much, drinks too much coffee, and works too hard, she says. With his black hair greased back, wearing tired polyester pants, he masks his nature, which his patients still see. They wait for hours in his office, which is so small that the crowd sometimes spills out onto the street. His nurses make frantic calls to the hospital, urging him to hurry; he smiles, responds, hangs up, apparently lost in the tempo set by the woman whose labor he is attending.

He lingers with couples after births, as if too much engaged to leave. He says the earthiest things to them; they beam, charged with fecundity, and only after they are calm does he wander over to his office, where he takes his patients in, one by one. Something he does makes them forget how long they have waited.

Penny says she thinks of him at night on the ward and how he's slow and graceful, like a black cat after midnight. He is deft, but when he must do brutal procedures, his explanation carries surrender in it. She thinks his patients must feel that he has joined with them in their sufferance of necessary pain. He must, because he sits with the bereaved.

Respecting Mike Szutowitz, vulnerable as his patients, we have to reconsider the idea that people's sex and/or their formal education make the difference in the way they perceive childbirth. Maybe a practitioner's personal inheritances precede those factors. Maybe their attitudes come from family and community. Mike's father, after all, was a general practitioner in a small town and may never have been estranged from his patients; perhaps Mike imitates him or, to put it another way, maybe he's got a feeling of village in his blood, like Zorba had dancing in his. Who knows what's innate and what's impressed?

Take Leo Sorger, an obstetrician who practices in Malden, Massachusetts. Trained in Germany, he learned to deliver women who were shaved, draped, and on their backs. It seemed, he says retrospectively, that the male physicians may have felt more comfortable with the woman well covered and with her body distorted by "forceps, spinals, tons of drugs." Then they did not have to think of the sexual implications of their work. Observing denuded parts, vulva and vagina only, they could lead themselves to think they were working on a "machine." When Sorger came to the States in the early sixties, he found the same shop atmosphere.

After he began practicing at the Malden Hospital, however, he encountered Elizabeth Noble, a well-known birth reformer and listened to her speak about the capability of women at birth. Was it because he was reminded of some births he'd attended out in the country in Germany, births where "I let the baby come out," that he heard her? Was it because he "came from a long line of craftsmen" that he grasped the possibilities of natural birth? Experimentally, cautiously, he gave up spinals and epidurals; eventually he bit the bullet and, in secret, attended a few home births. "I admired those women," he said. Ultimately, he changed his way of practice. When neighborhood women would come to his office, he told them he would be pleased to assist them either at home or at the office, but (excepting true necessity) there would be "no spinals, no episiotomies." He couldn't do those things anymore. They "repulsed" him.

Take David Gandel, the obstetrician practicing at Strong Memorial Hospital in Rochester, New York. When he says that he read Suzanne Arms's *Immaculate Deception* and was much moved by its "stinging, vitriolic" attack on obstetrics, one thinks he might have inherited some poetic blood; but then one hears that his mother died of complications of childbirth and suspects that he feels as he does because of that wound. But then we find out that he hung around a friend of a friend of Leboyer's, the French doctor who introduced the idea of "gentle birth" into childbirth circles and specifically identified birth as a "poetic experience." Maybe somebody guided him into his interest in psychology and psychosomatic medicine or maybe it was a genetic bent—his sister, after all, went into psychiatry. Did someone take him to Rush Medical College, a "unique institution"? And why did he take a year off from his training to travel in Europe and Africa, where he observed "how different cultures interpreted disease"? He must have had some feeling for women. He took the trouble to visit the cemetery in Rochester, Minnesota, where Susan B. Anthony is buried to "pay his respects."

The only thing we know for certain about David Gandel is that he is not narrowly educated. He knows some psychology (his undergraduate minor), has had anthropological thoughts, and is not unfamiliar with the status of women. So while he too toed the line during his residency, following the disease-oriented, do-something, pattern established there, once he went into practice on his own, "I decided to find my own way. I used techniques I had learned from midwives," e.g., walking, hot showers, choice in birth positions, and few episiotomies. He lowers lights and "hates" taking a patient to the delivery room.

Like midwives, he encounters women who are not keen on his philosophy. "American women are taught that having a baby is something to be frightened of," he says, anthropologically. Since they live in a "technologically dependent society," they manage their fear by "turning their bodies over to the obstetrician," but he approaches them in a noncontrolling way, he "tries to educate them," and some are "relieved when they find it can be another way." His patients "brag about not having episiotomies."

There's an appreciation of family life at the births he attends and there is a human, not institutional, mood. "These few moments are really special to the woman. The father often breaks down crying," and when a woman reaches out for her child after birth, strokes him, holds him, and looks into his eyes, Gandel says that the poet in him is satisfied.

Most doctors who break away from the strict medical management of birth have one thing in common: They have a breadth of experience. George Little, who took the leadership role in establishing a nurse-midwifery service at Dartmouth-Hitchcock Hospital, was exposed to midwifery as a medical student. He spent a couple of summers in a midwife-staffed hospital in Tanzania. "In fact, I can remember the person specifically," he says. "There was a Sister Leah, who was a Tanzanian and had been in the UK, and had trained in nurse-midwifery and headed up this small group of nurse-midwives." His experience initiated "a long-term interest in the role model." His mission for the maternal and child health department at Dartmouth-Hitchcock today is to combine the best of caring with the best of high tech.

His colleague Jack Dodds, the obstetrician, was also acquainted with midwifery early on his career. He "trained in Philadelphia. There were midwives in some situations and Booth [which had a midwifery-centered program] was one we helped to cover." His current midwife colleagues say that he is sometimes a better midwife than they are; he lets a woman push longer before he intervenes. Metaphorically speaking, "he smokes a longer cigar."

Wendy Savage studied epidemiology, infectious diseases, and sexual psychology, and she practiced in several cultures. Fredericka Heller had taken an advanced degree in history, had lived in Mexico for nine years, had married, had a child, and divorced. Valerie Jorgensen, the obstetrician who assists birth at the birthing suite at Pennsylvania Hospital, had taken an educational detour into psychiatry. Each of these practitioners has been exposed to dimensions of birthcare that are generally excluded by Western medicine, and they incorporate them in their practices. They may not be able to explain why such tolerances help birth any better than midwives can. Perhaps they just feel right and decent. But in each case the practitioner has relinquished some control, has made room for women, their families, and their beliefs. None fear calm and each has let a greater measure of life in. They teach us that safety need not be bought at the expense of humanity and they show us that birth is not just a physical affair, but a resounding moment in the life of a woman with child.

Labors of Midwives

If some doctors are prowling more human territory, one might imagine that midwives have gone the next step and are exploring that uncharted territory where mind and body swarm together; that they are proving the validity of the tenets of housewifery, the function of kindness and consideration in health, not to mention the spiritual advantages of the undisturbed birth.

Unfortunately, they have been otherwise occupied. As odd as it may seem—considering the fifty years of twentieth-century experience midwives have behind them—the profession is still getting its institutional walls up. Historically short of prestige and its associated advantages—time and money—midwives are still busy with survival issues. It's been all they could do to get schools established and students educated. It tells something about the status of the profession that the major publication of its college in the decade of the eighties is "Nurse-Midwifery in America,"[10] a report that describes who midwives are, how they are educated, how they practice, whether they are legal, helpful, and safe, etc. In other words, it's a tight, statistical identity document.

Their claims to safety and good care are founded on that very adequate but not very satisfying research we've mentioned. Joyce Thompson, CNM, knocking one basic professional chore out of the way, reviewed nurse-midwifery literature from 1925 to 1984. She summarizes: "The effectiveness of nurse-midwifery care was demonstrated repeatedly in various samples in various locations by increased use of services [which may only mean that women like it]. There was also a resultant decline in rates of maternal mortality, prematurity, and neonatal deaths [which is more promising]."[11] In other words, midwifery research has not unearthed the difficult proofs.

Thompson pats the profession on the head. "There is *some* [our emphasis] evidence that nurse-midwifery care is both safe and satisfying," and then she grabs it by the ear: "Now it is time to investigate the components of that care process and contribute to theory building and testing in nurse-midwifery. How does the way CNMs provide care during pregnancy differ from that of other providers? More important, do those differences contribute to better outcomes of care in terms of health and well-being of women and infants? If so, what is the relationship and which components can be replicated by other health professionals?"[12]

Does she hope that midwives will set out promptly to answer these questions? "Most CNMs are clinicians first and researchers last, if ever,"[13] she writes, somewhat balefully. Madeleine Shearer, the editor of the holistically oriented journal *Birth*, makes a similar assessment. "I don't see nurses and nurse-midwives doing much research. They are really doers, not researchers and writers. My view of it is that they aren't taught research, aren't taught the basic tenets of the scientific method. . . . They welcome research done by others, but they are unlikely to undertake it themselves."

Lack of predisposition, then, may be one factor that explains why midwives haven't been producing research papers, but another, much more likely, explanation is social and economic reality. Writing on the status of midwifery research in 1980, for example, an editorial in the *Journal of Nurse-Midwifery* says, "We have a limited number of nurse-midwives, who in turn have a limited number of hours which they can devote to their profession, not to mention the limitation of financial resources." Given these restrictions, she wonders rhetorically whether it's wise to divert energy into research. "What about the time and economics involved in seeking research grants, in carrying out the research design and in publishing the study?"[14]

Typical of 1988 is Lisa Sommers, a CNM practicing in Houston. She told us that she'd been wanting to write an article for the *Journal* on midwives who had gone on to get advanced degrees. She thought that her research findings might throw some light on the research future of the profession. It's been a year since she got the information together. "I haven't had time to write it," she said, citing her on-call schedule.

She, like her professional organization, will just have to get around to it when she can. Indeed, she might be comforted by their pace. It wasn't until 1987, after all, that the ACNM replaced its piddling $300 research budget with a not-exactly-spectacular one of $22,000. It's hoped that this money, invested in a pilot project, will attract outside money and help nurse-midwives as they establish a national data base—a system to count the number, place, and outcome of midwife-assisted births nationwide. In other words, the midwives are just getting the wiring in.

Not to paint too dark a picture, there are individual research projects going on. Some midwives with major institutions behind them have set out to make orderly proof of the midwife's contention that low-tech care is at least as good as, if not superior to, high-tech care. This back-to-the-future enterprise is based on one of medicine's oldest dictums, *primum non nocere,* which means "first, do no harm." The principle, as we have seen, is primary in midwifery—robust in its suspicion of intervention, which medicine, as we have seen, has rushed to embrace. Indeed, in medicine, technical interventions tend to be rashly taken up and used widely *before* their worth has been adequately demonstrated. Anne Oakley, a highly respected historian of birth practices, mentions X rays, inductions, and ultrasound as examples of this historical pattern. But the list could go on: scopolamine, episiotomies, fetal monitoring, and routine hospitalization, for example.

In the past, midwives have expressed their disagreement with the overzealous interventionists by carping at obstetricians and hospitals. Today, Lisa Paine, a certified nurse-midwife working on her doctorate in public health at Johns Hopkins University, is systematically comparing the accuracy of listening to the baby with a fetoscope (stethoscope) as opposed to the electronic fetal monitor while doing nonstress tests. (Nonstress tests are done to assess the baby's vitality.)[15] In a similar *primum non nocere* project, Joyce Roberts at the University of Colorado is evaluating birth positions: Do babies do better if their mothers are in the high-tech lithotomy position or in the low-tech squatting, standing, kneeling postures?[16]

At Columbia University, Betty Carrington, EdD, CNM, is looking into the accuracy of low-tech methods—that is, using hands and measuring tape—in comparison to ultrasound for estimating a baby's birth weight while a mother is laboring, in order to prepare optimally for birth.[17]

The experiments may sound retrograde, but there's intelligence operating here. If midwives can establish when stethoscope, hands, and measuring tape work well, then fewer women will have to undergo those testing procedures that undercut their confidence in their bodies. They may be able to avoid the physical and emotional risks of certain technical procedures.

So a few midwives with some well-heeled institutions behind them are beginning to prove in that necessary, systematic fashion that their methods are reliable. To do so, of course, they must assume the unloved task of challenging some of the habits of medical science. And while it seems unfortunate that so much midwifery labor must be committed to undoing what has been done and while one is tempted to complain that medical science should have figured out what simple measures worked before they started up with the complicated ones, there's no point. The proofs are needed.

Besides, high tech can be a midwife's ally. Not just in saving those women and babies who have genuine obstetrical complications, but also in research. Joyce Roberts, mentioned above, has used intrauterine pressure catheters to measure contractions and is taking cord blood samples to read the Ph of a baby's blood. As Lisa Paine comments, "We are using high-tech methods to investigate the benefits of low-tech."

More profoundly, high tech is doing scientific service—if unintentionally—by defining its limits. We might not have appreciated the value of the "qualified labor room personnel" had they not been shown to be equal or superior to the fetal monitor for monitoring labor. High tech may even prompt us to ask whether human care has added value. And if so, why?

Thus we find ourselves right back to the unanswered questions we raised when we were reviewing Varney's *Nurse-Midwifery.* What's the value of less interventive, more down-to earth care? How do we show that fluffy pillows, nice touching, and compassionate listening make a difference? And who is to undertake the incredibly complex task of demonstrating that the way a woman feels, the way she is treated, the environment she is in, can affect the course of her birth? We are so ill equipped to study mind-body relationships. Who dares to prove the axioms of housewifery?

A Few

Valerie Hodenius, CNM, a big chortling woman, cannot stop herself from telling birth stories. "I had a friend," she says right off the bat, "who had a ten-pound baby [the first time]. . . . She was also a psychologist so she was into 'Yes, the head and the uterus have some connection; they're not totally separate'—like when our periods are late when we're under stress." The friend had come to Valerie for her second baby, ready to have it on her own.

"She goes into labor. . . . She goes to nine centimeters [dilated], and she's at nine and she's at nine and she's at nine and she won't finish," Valerie said, punctuating the stalled labor. Since there weren't any apparent physical problems, Valerie asked her, "What's cooking?"

And her friend said, "I don't want this baby to come out and disappear." Valerie asked her why she was thinking that, and her friend began talking about how she was adopted and how she was lost to her biological mother and her biological mother was lost to her and "then [she] went into an hour of sobbing and healing and having feelings about being given up for adoption." When that emotional storm passed, "Boom! Out comes this twelve-and-a-half-pounder.

"In a different institution," Valerie went on, "she would have been sectioned and everyone would have said, 'Ooooh. That [the section] is legitimate. Look at this huge baby; of course she couldn't give birth to it.' " But Valerie, who has an undergraduate degree in psychology and who has maintained an interest in the subject, had an entirely different opinion. "She couldn't [give birth] until she finished that processing."

She is fierce on the subject. "What I've found is that when women stop their labor and get into this failure to progress or dysfunctional labor, ninety-nine times out of a hundred there is something that a woman needs or wants to do. Sometimes it can be just 'Leave me alone, I want to sleep and then I can carry on'. . . . But sometimes they do powerful things."

Once again, she threw herself into a story. "I had another woman who had had a cesarean with a good physician who had let her labor and labor and labor and push and push and the kid never went into the pelvis. [Now she's pregnant with her] second baby. She wants a vaginal birth."

When the woman went into labor, everything was "normal, average." Then it stalled. "A few piddling contractions . . . " The woman, apparently searching for companionship in labor, asked Valerie to tell her birth stories. "So I tell her my birth stories and that didn't fix it." They moved into their experiences of love and loving. "She tells me her story with her husband who had been a priest and

. . . the difficulty they went through coming together. That didn't fix it." Stuck herself, but trusting the emotional undercurrents of labor to carry the woman through, Valerie sent her and her husband out of the hospital to have some dinner. When they came back, the woman said, "When I was a kid I was physically abused."

"Yeah."

"I was beaten on the head."

"Yeah."

"I'm afraid of hurting my baby's head."

Valerie worked two angles. She reassured the woman that birth was good for babies, it stimulated them and prepared them to grab onto life outside. At the same time, she taught her that the pain of childbirth was not arbitrary and capricious—as those childhood beatings had seemed to be—they were a result of her body's work. She "gave" control of pain to the woman. "This is your pain. When you want to make a contraction, you make one. I want you to only make it as big as you want it to be. . . . This is yours."

Within a couple of hours she was "whipping out these whopping contractions . . . and just kept making them and birthed her baby."

For Valerie, for Lisa Sommers, and for many nurse-midwives in the United States today, birth is a process of interplay between body and soul. It's a snapshot of a woman's state of being, a product of her personal history, her culture, her dreams, and her nightmares. It is an opportunity for healing past injuries and ripe with potential for inner growth, the kind that will nourish transformation into motherhood. It is here, these women say, with the remarriage of mind and body, that our most fruitful research into birth will be done. That is, as soon as we find out how to do it.

The Holistic Inquiry

Enter then, the adventurous holists, those health theorists willing to consider unorthodox connections between mind and body. "Holistic prenatal care may appear doomed to frustration from its inception," Lewis Mehl and Gayle Peterson admit in *Pregnancy as Healing*. "How can we consider everything? How do sunspots affect birth? Is astrology important? How does the experience of anxiety about combining motherhood and career . . . affect birth?"[18]

They ask the questions anyway, unembarrassed by the seeming absurdity of their questions or the sure absence of answers to them. "In a holistic approach," they write, "we are interested in anything that works, even if we can't explain how or why it works,"[19] and in this way they challenge the biomedical model of birth which, they say, is too mechanical and narrow, too exclusive. It mistakenly isolates birth from women and women from their environment.

They say that the human, birthing or not, is by definition an organism in relationship to the environment. The human is perpetually in flux, its inner state adapting to its outer. "All parts of the psyche, including the body, are always striving towards an integration and an increased level of cooperation in living."[20] We may think that our misperformances—like birth complications, for example— are evidence of some shameful internal inadequacy, but by holistic standards, that's not so. Just as "health is a dynamic and creative balance of energy," so "disease is a form of healing. It is the body's attempt to alter or bring into perspective the mind's experience of the world."[21] All we ever do in the holistic state is adjust inner to outer conditions. It gets hot, we sweat; it gets dangerous, we run or fight back. Therefore, we err when we judge our bodies (or our subconscious) to be good or bad, successful or failing; better to respect our internal intelligence. A person is no more "perfect" in health than "imperfect" in disease. A woman is no more "right" to have a normal birth than "wrong" to experience complications. Complications, whether present or absent, are simply expressions of that constant readjustment we make in our striving toward integration.

But if everyone is already doing what they are supposed to be doing—i.e., naturally and constantly striving toward resolution of stress—then one might wonder why the holists bring up the subject of intervention at all. If the body will adapt to circumstances in its own good way, then why shouldn't the caregiver adopt a laissez-faire attitude toward birth?

The answer rests on the assumption that humans are as much a part of one another's environment as sun and rain. The caregiver's behavior, before, during, and after a woman's birth, is a factor in the niche. The doctor, the midwife, the nurse, the partner are inevitably part of the outer state. Thus Odent created a physical environment at Pithiviers, but he also created a psychological one when he kept his distance. Penny introduced an alternative physical environment when she sent that young couple down to the creek, but also suggested that they learn to depend on one another.

The woman who hears from mother, friends, neighbors, doctors, and hospital that she should take drugs at birth is in a specific and limited intellectual and emotional environment. Certainly her inner state may cause her to reject this solution—maybe she's a recovering addict and harbors a fear of drugs, maybe she's got an earthy propensity, maybe she's read that in other places women give birth without drugs, maybe she has a powerful need to rebel against the prevailing custom—but her choice is constrained by the information and services available to her and it is dramatically influenced by the prevailing beliefs of those around her.

The job of the holist, then, is to help a woman clarify her thinking about her inner state. Does she want drugs at birth because she recognizes her need to belong to a community and thus to follow its prescribed patterns? Or does her informational environment convince her that drugs are best? Does she want drugs at birth because she feels she is "not good with pain"? Or does she want drugs at birth because she doesn't know how to resolve the anticipated stress any other way? If it is the latter, then the holists, in that ecumenical spirit of theirs, may introduce other choices into her personal and cultural niche.

So Peterson and Mehl counsel women during their pregnancies. Like obstetricians and midwives, they are interested in identifying factors that indicate a woman might have complications at birth, but at that point the similarity diffuses. They recognize the medical importance of hypertension, for example, but they also think about what hypertension tells about a woman's life state and ways of coping. How does it solve stress problems for her? Which stress problems does it solve? What other ways might they be solved?

Peterson and Mehl throw in everything they can think of. What's a woman's relationship to her body? Does she trust it? Does she listen to it? What's her relationship to her partner? Under what circumstances does she depend upon him or her and vice versa? What are their attitudes toward the birth? Did anyone in their families die giving birth? What were their mothers' stories? What does the woman value in life? What kind of birth does she want? Why? What psychosocial circumstances enable her to trust herself and her body; which deter her? They ask all these questions because they believe it is not one factor that determines the outcome of a birth but the infinite interplay of factors. "Holistic prenatal care requires the discovery of how variables are synthesized to create a whole."[22]

As a woman understands her inner state, the holists say, she can make a better choice from her outer state. Suppose that a woman is an athlete and that she has learned how to control the ticking of her smallest muscles. Suppose she learns that what is good for competition—i.e., utmost control—is not particularly beneficial to birth, which enjoys surrender. Given this information about her body, she can actively select an environment that encourages her to let go. One woman athlete, for example, labored most effectively when her birth companions stayed with her, massaged her, and held her. It seemed that their participation relieved her of some of the responsibility she felt for her body.

Another woman, by contrast, preferred to be directed rather than to control. Her primary adaptation was to set aside her inner urgings and to do as others suggested. The style seemed to serve her in life, but it was troublesome in labor. She would labor well when left alone, but when a nurse or midwife entered the room, she would shut off her body's instructions and ask, "What do I do now?"—a transference of control that tended to cause her labor to slow. Her caregivers found that they helped her most when they left her undisturbed.

Holists, in other words, do not propose a set behavior for the woman or for those who are with her at birth. They attempt to understand what kind of attention or intervention might be best for a particular woman in a particular circumstance and, like the midwives, take continual instruction from whatever works.

What works, they say, is the body and mind together. Like Michael Odent, like the psychoneuroimmunologists, like Wendy Savage, like some obstetricians, like some midwives, and, no doubt, like some of those "qualified labor room personnel," they find that what a woman thinks and feels and how she relates to her environment dramatically affect the course of her birth. In order to develop more effective interventions, they continue to follow the hormonal and behavioral trails that might explain some of these connections. At the same time, they do not expect, ever, to prescribe a labor pattern. They do not anticipate being in control. "We are forever *uncertain,"* they write. "Since the universe as a whole can affect [a woman], and, we, as a part, can never fully grasp the whole, we can never fully predict what will happen to [her]."[23]

PART IV

COMPENSATING FOR THE LOSS

Introduction

P ETERSON AND Mehl's book is called *Pregnancy as Healing.* Healing implies that there has been a wound or disease. It suggests that American woman may need to recover from subtle reproductive injury in order to give birth, that they require intricate psychological attention.

We were back in Penny's living room when we discussed Peterson and Mehl. While we talked, we looked out over fields of corn and hay lapping in the weather, saw the horses, released from the barn, charge for the meadow and, intermittently, watched the cows shamble about the pasture. Children came up the lane in the morning, lunch pails banging their knees. Horses and buggies rattled into view, raising dust; their riders got out and greeted the dog, who slavered on their hands. The wash was strung out on long lines and flapped ebulliently over lawn and garden.

From Penny's window, the earth is bountiful. The land is all soft bellies, mounded breasts, and broad hips. The dirt itself is plump. So provocative is this landscape that the otherwise emotionally restrained Amish seem to make love to her, feed her, braid her tidy rows, let them unravel out, leave her pastures to rest, rotate her crops. The Amish are careful not to compliment one another, but they lavish praise on nature—they comment on shadows thrown by trees and on the flitting of lavender moths. By a slight gesture, they touch the sky at sunset, which is the rosy color of fresh-bathed white skin. The earth is Rubenesque and the Amish relish her.

The person who cares for pregnant Amish women seldom needs to do intricate emotional work. Little healing is called for. Rarely must there be elaborate psychological schemes. The women come to their prenatal checkups and later on they have their babies. Apparently Amish women are adequately nourished, both physically and emotionally, for giving birth. Apparently they carry fewer reproductive wounds.

It is reasonable, we thought, looking down over the land, so well nourished and unwounded. The Amish, who are considered to be among the finest farmers in the world, live intimately with the land, they depend upon her, they stroke her, handle her dirt, and plant some of her crops by hand. For three centuries they have worked this land and it is said to get richer, more fecund every year. They have a legacy, passed from generation to generation: It says that if you treat the land well, it will reproduce well; it you neglect it, it will not.

Women birth as they live, Peterson writes in another book, *Birthing Normally* (1981). If American women are so often wounded at birth, then they must be wounded also in life. If they distrust their bodies at birth, then they have learned to distrust them.

Which means that we, as a people, must have lost our knowledge of how to care for the reproductive lives of women. We must be neglecting them. Just as we seem to have lost our sensitivity to Mother Nature, we seem to have lost our sensitivity to Mother. We do not relish her. We do not provide. If we did, the subject of healing would be less likely to come up.

Mothering

WANTING TO control the danger and pain of the birth process, we invented medicalized management. It had unexpected and unfortunate side effects: It ended women's reign of decision-making in the birthplace and, in a Machiavellian turn, prevented women from experiencing the power of birth for herself. It also distorted the process of birth. For decades, indeed, up to the present, neither doctors nor women have been able to distinguish between the complications that medicine was causing (iatrogenic) and those that erupted naturally from women's bodies. In an era in which science was more credited than women, the benefit of the doubt went to science. Thus individual women like Sheryl felt that something was wrong with them when their babies had problems, and the troublesome outcomes perpetuated the impression in women that their bodies were untrustworthy. They submitted even more to medical management.

Caretakers, observing women's submissive posture, came to think of birthing women as nonpowerful persons and treated them accordingly, which further diminished women's self-esteem. Over time, some practitioners and, to an extent, the profession itself developed a feeling of contempt for the weakened women. Thus the casualness of huge episiotomies and seesawing forceps.

Being abused, women adopted the mentality of victims and were more likely to be further abused.

In Amish culture, women avoided the medicalization craze and continued to believe in themselves as birthers. Not to say that they have been impervious to technology—many Amish women have employed physicians and hospitals, but that generally was a temporary function of the marketplace. Only when they couldn't find anyone to attend them at home would they go to the hospital.

As a result, the legacy of birth was never completely lost. Enough young women remember how their mothers' bellies went from large to bursting, remember how, one evening, without much fuss, they were taken to their grandmothers' houses and how, the next morning, they returned to find their mothers' bellies down and a new baby in the house. The message that traveled from mother to daughter was that birth was another kind of work a woman did and that it was best to get on with it.

Young Amish women expect to give birth. It isn't something to be proven, as in, "We'll just see how you do," it just happens, like lambing, like spring, summer, winter, and fall. For the Amish, the rhythms of nature are not exceptional, like a weekend in the country, but the daily stuff of their lives.

This attunement to nature may supersede all other factors in their lives. It deeply influences the way they treat each other, which is similar to the way they treat the land—by stewardship and with an eye on the long term. Each member of the community, male and female, is respected, not because it is written up as the way people should behave, but because it is essential to the community's survival.

Visitors to Amish country often miss the gender respect prevailing in Amish society. What they pick up are the signs of rigid, sex-specific roles. They see that a girl is raised to run the home and that a boy is raised to run the farm. They see that she learns to cook, clean, sew, set the table, quilt, wash the dishes, plant the garden, write letters, have babies, and tend them. On the side, by selling her quilts or shoofly pies or bread in a shop or stand, she brings in a little cash. Visitors remark on how unliberated these poor women are.

A boy, oblivious to urban measurements of equality, rarely clears the table or washes a dish. He'll turn the garden with a cultivator, and maybe help plant, but you won't find him helping with the preserving. Instead, he repairs harnesses, solders broken equipment, calculates the returns from milk sales, goes to the bank, hardware store, and any necessary public meetings. His sister stays home and puts a fresh coat of white paint on the windowframe. When the boys are in their teens, and before they join the church, they might sample bars, cars, and the Wild West in a van with their friends. Girls are adventurous if they go to the Jersey shore with girlfriends and rent a bicycle. A girl waits for a boy to pick her out of a gaggle of girls at Sunday supper and ask her if she would be willing to ride home in his buggy with him. She can say no then or later if she finds she doesn't care for him, but she is not free to initiate a relationship herself.

One set of rules for the women, another set of rules for the men, and the enforcement methods are compelling. If one steps out of line, one finds oneself bypassed at quiltings or left alone at the horse auction.

For all the strict gender-typing, however, it is a mistake to think of Amish females as being lesser. Among these people, women are highly valued, not only for their daily labor but specifically because they are of the mothering sex. Penny's experience with a young couple, Manuel and Suzie, shows how it works.

Mothering the Mother

I couldn't figure out why Manuel would have married Suzie. Manuel reminds me of my cousin Rod, which is to say he's a warm, tousled animal. I see Manuel and I think how Rod, even today, will grab me by my waist and pull me down into his capacious lap after dinner, just like he did when he was an officer in the navy and I was an ogle-eyed, infatuated six-year-old. Contrary to all rules of growth, my shoulder slips just as cozily into his armpits as it ever did. His animal snuggling comes as naturally to him as restoring houses, making money, or roaring, great-balls-of-fire, in his beat-up car with his family to get double-decker ice creams. You can't be depressed with Rod around, because if something goes wrong, he has so much fun fixing it up.

Manuel's the same. One fall day a few years after I came out to the County, I was scraping paint off the front door. I had a string of deliveries, a batch of family demands, and I was feeling resentful about never having any time for myself: For every free hour I claimed, there were a dozen household chores to catch up on. Anyway, I'd just begun my lackluster effort to prepare the door for painting when I heard the crunching of buggy wheels on my driveway. I felt like crying. I knew some Amishman wanted something from me and I knew I had nothing left to give.

Manuel jumped out of the buggy, then reached back in and pulled out his two-year-old nephew Johnny, whom he slung under his arm like a sack of fodder. Johnny hung there, grinning foolishly. Manuel sauntered over, the child under his arm, took the scraper from my hand, cruised it up and down the door, and ten minutes later the job was done. Now beholden, I felt only slightly more hospitable.

So when Manuel wondered if I remembered what day it was I folded my arms and waited wearily for the rest to come: The Amish will just be wondering if you would be going into town. Only after you waffle out that response and gerrymander your way through the answers to a couple more off-the point questions do you find out that somebody wants a ride to visit their sister Martha who sort of lives in that direction or that there's a genuine emergency and someone needs a ride to the hospital. You can't evade the process because you never know if something important is behind it.

Since I failed to recall the significance of the day, Manuel explained, with a Rod-like twinkle in his eye, that it was exactly a year ago today that his and Suzie's Matthew had been born and they just thought maybe I'd like to come down to their house for cake and ice cream (and pretzels and chips and cookies and weather talk and I would be "on," answering baby questions from the assembled women). Now that my door was scraped, I couldn't really say no; nor could I tell Manuel how hard it was for me to visit his Suzie.

When I first saw her I thought she was one of a small number of Amish "princesses." Usually the oldest daughter, they must assume authority over their brothers and sisters at an early age. By the time they get to me, and because they've carried the burden of that authority for many years, they sometimes treat me like a rumpled sister. To them, I'm a fumbler, a person whom they have to see, because it is ordered, but hardly necessary for women like themselves. I wait, not challenging them, because I've learned that birth will teach them what I never could: that a baby can't be born against pride. It holds the muscles too stiff and the backbone too straight.

Suzie was particularly arrogant. In no uncertain terms, she let me know that she hadn't chosen me as her caregiver. In her family, she said tartly, women employed doctors and had their babies in hospitals. But Manuel had wanted her to come to me, his sisters had, his mother recommended it, and so here she was, suffering the indignities of wifehood. She seemed little moved by the child moving within her and mentioned several times that "Manuel had no idea of how uncomfortable it was." That man, unperturbed, ministered to her without fail.

I'd stand in the doorway of the examining room when we were done and watch her slip out of the office, leaving Manuel behind to check out a paperback from our birth library. I'd glance at the title to see what questions he'd bring the next time, and then glance out the window at her, sitting with head held uncomfortably high in the carriage. I shook my head and muttered, "C-section."

I fought with myself over this prognosis, which in fact had no physiological basis. It was more like a scent I picked up from Suzie, for whom pregnancy seemed to be an imposition, something she, as an Amish wife, had to do but for which she was not prepared. As it turned out, she wasn't the same as the other princesses, who had an idea that they could have a baby without mussing the sheets. Suzie was pronouncing, "I won't do it your way"; what she meant was, "I can't."

I couldn't decide what to do. On the one hand, I knew that if she didn't believe she could give birth on her own, she wouldn't. A midwife friend of mine calls it the "baby-no-come-out syndrome." If a woman doesn't feel that it's safe to have her baby, she'll withhold it. If we proceeded with home birth plans and if Suzie continued to resist, we'd end up with an emergency trip to the hospital and probably that cesarean, which would just make things worse.

On the other hand, Suzie, like it or not, was going to have several babies and, what's more, she had a lifetime of mothering ahead of her. She needed every hormonal and human advantage we could ply her with. If we sent her to the hospital, it might solve the immediate problem of getting the baby out, but it would not serve her greater life need—which was to discover, for herself, her own generative capacities.

And then there was Manuel. Manuel, like Rod, arms open, lap warm, itching for family to clamber in and on. So I fussed extravagantly when Suzie came into the office. I asked what she thought about the childbirth classes. I showed her pictures of the developing fetus. I talked to her about her quilting, of which she was proud. I admired the color of her dress. I gave her some flannel so she could make sleepers for the baby. I made lame excuses to stop by her house, thinking it might help if she got used to seeing me there. It was, as you might suspect, immaculate. Never a glass in the sink, never a wrinkle on the bedcovers. The wood paneling had been painted and appeared to be waxed. A brand new, beautifully crafted baby's cradle was installed not in its parents' room but in the bedroom adjoining.

Suzie was never alone when I visited. Her mother-in-law would be sitting in the rocking chair stitching patches on a jacket, a cousin would be in the summer kitchen screwing the tops of canning jars tight, a neighbor would be at the quilting frame, or an aunt nursing her newborn on the couch. While Suzie moved stiffly among these women as if they were handmaidens, they carried on, evenly humming, through their communal housewifery.

A week before the baby was due, I saw Suzie at a wedding. We women were lined up on long benches after the meal was over and after the men had stepped outdoors to lean against the carriages and gossip. The women passed their babies back and forth, cooing at them, letting them drowse in their arms, and we babbled about raking leaves, who'd had twins, how Becca's husband was recovering from that throw from a horse. Suzie, who was seated about halfway down the row, right between the mother of an infant and a woman who was quite pregnant herself, got more than her share of baby-passing. The first time a child landed on her, I saw her start. Her arms stuck out stiff, like blades on a plow, and soon the baby began to cry. Her neighbor, the mother of the child, reached over and resettled the child in Suzie's arms. "He's always fussy in that position," she said. "He likes to have his head just so," and she cradled Suzie's arms to show her.

"It'll be harder for her," the woman next to me said, "being as she won't have her mother to help her."

"Why would that be?" I said, pretending, as one is supposed to do, that I wasn't curious.

"Why? Didn't you know, Penny?"

"Why no, I didn't."

"Her mother died when she was eight and her father didn't marry again until just last year. Elam Stoltfus's widow? From Perry County? Did you know them?" We worked out that I didn't and we hastened to other topics, but I'd been informed that Suzie had been without a mother during her adolescent years. From that, I knew that she didn't know how to change a diaper, avoid a breast infection, take a temperature, strain vegetables, make up baby clothes, and so on.

The way the women on the bench surrounded Suzie, it was the Amish answer to the problem of the incapacitated mother: Other women gathered around her. Like when Lizzie, mother of seven, was confined to bed for the last four months of her pregnancy. Although she never stopped working—she braided rugs, snapped beans, peeled potatoes, did hand sewing for the neighborhood, planned the meals, and combed the kids' hair during her confinement—she could not run her house and so, while she lay in bed, other women streamed evenly through her kitchen and out into the garden. Never breaking rhythm, the clothes got hung out, the floor washed, the dishes done, the casseroles, pies, and cakes made. Lizzie's husband got the older kids ready for school, the younger ones traipsed around after him during the day, and he prayed and bedded them at night. When a woman's ability to work was interrupted, others took it up.

Since Suzie's knowledge of motherhood was insufficient, the women sifted into the void, as inevitably as sand slides into a hole. They appeared in her kitchen, keeping her company, mothering her, showing her how babies were held and nursed and bathed and cuddled. Manuel paraded sample children past her. His brother had crafted that cradle. Her people, never speaking of it, brought the mothering legacy to her door. They trained her with the padding of their feet on the kitchen floor, with the rhythm of their work, and by the steady, telling patterns of their lives.

Suzie labored in a halting fashion for forty-eight hours. She stalled at four centimeters and didn't start up again until her mother-in-law came over and massaged her feet. Manuel, not missing one of her cues, came and went as she needed. Only when I'd exhausted my repertoire of support measures did she begin to push, which she also resisted. And then, at the last minute, she cried out, "Make it stop," and the baby did, one short push away from birth.

I had only one trick left. I told her we would wait until she decided to have her baby. I consciously relaxed myself, elbow on her knee, and stared out the window. Manuel sat meditatively, hands in his lap. It took her about three minutes to give herself up to reality, whereupon I felt the tremors of a determined contraction rolling through her and, as suddenly, the baby was out and in my hands.

When she glimpsed the child, she started, as if shocked by what she had produced. I put him on her stomach and she arched her back. Then Manuel moved in, smoothing her hair, mumbling in Pennsylvania Dutch, and as soon as the cord was cut he picked up the child, wrapped him, walked him around while Suzie delivered her placenta, and then he placed the baby at her side. He sat himself down too, his back touching her knee, and he began to stroke the two of them as if they were still one. When Suzie reached one finger toward Matthew's ear, I left the room. When I returned, the baby was at her breast.

Suzie didn't become a great mother. She yanks Matthew's diaper too tight, she brushes his hair with a hard brush and disciplines him with a rigor beyond his age. When he gets sick, she seems paralyzed, and her mother-in-law has to take over the nursing. But she's always aware of him, she picks him up when he cries, nurses him, and does seem to enjoy dressing him up in his little trousers, which she learned to make from a neighbor. At that birthday party, which I did attend, she didn't scoop him up adoringly, as Manuel did, cake frosting and all, but when he got tired she lifted him out of Manuel's arm and affectionately carried him off to bed.

I learned from the Amish that mothering can be thought of as essential work. One that's worthy of community effort. True, it's easier for them than it is for families in the mainstream. Most Amish men and women work at home; grandparents live nearby and hands join conveniently; they don't have to raise their children to be free-standing in an unpredictable society; and they have the luxury of a slowly changing social order. They know they will live together for a lifetime and that the baby who is born today will be doing his mother's chores for her when she is old.

But for all that, theirs is a choice, a matter of priorities. As a people, they have chosen to value family. The importance placed on mothering work follows from that choice. It is as important to them as bringing in the harvest or getting the milking done. If the usual person can't do it, then somebody else takes up the responsibility. Mothering, regardless of who does it, is honored work. Like so many things here, it's the simplicity that knocks you over.

Unmothered Mothers

As long as humankind can remember, birth has been a moment of binding among women. For centuries, women have caught one another's children, breathed welcome on them, palmed their buttocks, and passed life on. Tiny, pathetic, pouched and blotched things, the new ones. Demanding our protection, they inspire us individually and renew us communally. With infants in our arms, we want nothing more than that they should live.

Perhaps it is only nature, with purposes independent of our own, that makes us respond with such clear purpose; nature that has issued the order that each species have an irresistible urge to survive. Nature, using unthinkable weaponry—sexual desire—which drives us to exhausting searches for partners with whom we might copulate. Nature, exploding in us a lust to bear a child. Nature that makes the smell of a newborn mesmerizing. Nature that makes us captive of a child for life.

Until very recently, women have been unable to avoid the reproductive imperative. There would be children, and women—who
could suckle them and who had learned nurturing skills at their
mothers' side—would raise them. The human responsibilities were
unending, and women made alliances among themselves to meet
them. "Dearest mother mine," women used to write, expecting their
mothers' companionship for their "great emergency" and also for the
ordeal of rearing children. Young women drew on the experience
and assistance of their mothers, sisters, aunts, cousins, and neighbors.

With the advent of mid-twentieth-century feminism, however, the
legacy of motherhood, like the legacy of birth, suffered a hatchet
blow. The mothers of today's mothers, the ones who, like centuries
of women before them, would teach their daughters how to meet
their reproductive obligation, were criticized for the patterns they
had made. The very themes they lived by—selflessness, tireless labor,
and subservience—led too often to self-destruction. Daughters
looked at their mothers, at their losses, their silences, their slow
deaths by self-abnegation, and thought of them as situational ene-
mies. Surely individual women still loved their individual mothers or
hated them or some of both, but in a cultural sense, the mothers'
lives, so filled with drudgery and repetition, and, most painfully,
disrespect, were not models for their daughters' lives, but their an-
tithesis.

"My mother never had herself," one professional woman told us
somberly. "She only had her kids. . . . She was dependent." Another,
determined that it wouldn't be the same for her, said that her mother
was of the "generation of women who are very bitter. Who stayed
home because that's what they did and didn't really feel like they
were capable of working. Who resented it. Who resented raising their
kids." Another interrupted her description of her own pleasure with
her child to say, as if still stunned by the news, "I just discovered
how unhappy my mother was when I was growing up."

Feminists called attention to all the ways in which women's lives
had been eaten up by the tasks of regeneration. Simone de Beauvoir
said that the fetus invades our bodies and then feeds like a parasite
on it. The woman may possess the infant, but she is also "possessed

by it . . . she feels herself tossed and driven, the plaything of obscure forces." She is "the prey of the species." When the fields needed hands, women had to deliver them; when war depopulated, women had to replace; while men were away, women had to shepherd the flock. Never mind women's imaginations, curiosities, or talents.

"To Simone de Beauvoir and others," Hester Eisenstein writes in her 1984 book, *Contemporary Feminist Thought,* "the mammalian [i.e., reproductive] responsibility of women was that difference that most condemned women to an unfree existence."[1] It was motherhood that leached life out of a woman, restrained her, kept her small, undeveloped, and out of sight. It was motherhood that kept women down, tied them to the house, motherhood that made them passive before men, that turned women's brains to mush, distracted them from reading, thinking, writing, painting, politicking, traveling, making money, gaining power. It was motherhood paradoxically, that kept them from rejoicing in their children—who, so innocent-eyed, were also the keepers of the prison.

The very axiom of the sixties liberation movement, Eisenstein says, was that feminism and motherhood were in "diametrical opposition." Many members of the movement chose to be childless and "motherhood—the bearing and raising of children—seemed to be rather more a barrier to self-fulfillment in women than a vehicle for it."[2] Beating the argument to the thin extreme, insisting that women must be known as free before they would be considered equal, the feminist Shulamith Firestone argued that reproduction of the species should be engineered.

The antireproductive mind-set, although promoted by a minority of women, invaded our culture. Women, imagining lives not consumed by family, found that circumstances permitted them to go ahead and invent them. Because of technological changes, one didn't have to slave eighteen hours a day just to keep a home together; because of affluence, more women might get educations; because of the civil rights movement, women could believe in equal opportunity for all.

In reproductive matters, obligatory childbearing was terminated. First there was the harbinger—the tampon, which freed women from the messy evidence of their mammalian nature—and then came free flight: the revolutionary contraceptive pill, which a woman could take without consultation with anyone and which allowed her to indulge in intercourse without the harrowing fear of unwanted pregnancy. If contraception failed, she could have an abortion, safely and legally. The hysterectomy, the removal of the offending uterus, became one of our most popular surgeries.

In the years during which today's childbearing women were growing up, educated women were not only able to forget the old imperatives of reproduction, they were also encouraged to dismiss the emotional content of sex. The *Cosmo* girl—urban, leggy, cleavaged, glamorous, and free—was to take sexual partners as men did, without fore- or afterfeeling. An abortion was a rational choice, and there was a mood suggesting it could and sometimes should be accomplished without emotional disruption. Living together was promoted for its sexual convenience. Having babies, especially in the early years of one's career, was questionable, not only because it interfered with one's professional climb but because it hampered one's free exploration of self and world. In fact, being deeply involved with children at any time tended to be a sign either of simplemindedness or outright betrayal of the movement. Magazines carried stories and photographs of enviable women who wore abbreviated ties and tailored suits.

The historic assignment given to young women growing up in the *Feminine Mystique* years was a staggering one: They were to revolutionize the centuries-old patterns of female behavior, not only by performing in the "real world" but also by destroying the roots of women's bondage: her motherhood.

The women's success has been phenomenal. Imitating the discipline that career-minded males follow, women committed themselves to long hours and single-purpose work. Leaving aside, as the men did, concern with domestic issues, they established their worth with astonishing speed. It was exactly as the feminists had said: Give women equal opportunity and they will perform equally. And while our culture drags more slowly than many of us would like in accepting the fact, while the number of women in positions of great power is still meagre, while subtle repressions abound and sexual harassment in the workplace continues, none of these transitional obstacles contradict the now irrefutable fact that women can be able lawyers, doctors, business people, artists, and politicians. A clear, clean, and irreversible demonstration was made.

In the same period of time—roughly from the mid-sixties to the mid-eighties, birth practices show a peculiar pattern. In the early years of liberation, birth reform caught on. The woman who had a baby naturally was thought to be accepting her personal power and showing her pride in her womanhood. In 1970 one Judy Potter, we remember, was arguing anti–sex discrimination law for the Equal Employment Opportunity Commission when she took a moment off to have her first child. Having threatened the medical personnel with a lawsuit if they so much as touched her, she had her baby unbothered.

Feminists rebelled against the "Immaculate Deception" of the medicalized birth and defended the right to have midwives. Women marched on The Yale Green in the mid-seventies, for example, to protest the closing of a midwifery service at Yale. Employing their consumer power, they insisted on less medicalized environments for labors. Decorators hung curtains in labor rooms and some out-of-hospital birth centers opened.

Then, say the elders of midwifery, women like Ruth Wilf, Kitty Ernst, and Charlotte Houde, enthusiasm waned. They say that birth is worse, more medicalized, than it ever was. Most are at a loss to explain the evolution; they get stuck with the paradox: Why do so many self-reliant women choose to be passive at birth?

What has been overlooked is the influence of the workplace, which, being male, has little systemic sympathy for reproduction. Women who wished to succeed did so by behaving as men did—at first by keeping sex emotionally unencumbered and then by keeping pregnancy, birth, and childrearing out of sight and out of mind. The course of a woman's pregnancy, formerly leavened by a klatch of buzzing women, was to be as close to invisible as one could make it.

Carol, for example, is now a witty, enthusiastic mother of four.

Her blond hair bobs like a golden apple when she laughs, which she does often, adding yet another wry bit to her collection of stories on the life of the suburban mother. By our reckoning, Carol must have been about nine years old when the *Feminine Mystique* was published. By the time she was twenty-five, she'd aced the assignment given to her generation. She had a job in publishing in New York, was meeting famous people, taking long lunches in chic restaurants, and generally living the much-advertised, glamorous life. She was married and then, rather prematurely, got pregnant. "I was working . . . in a managerial job and in the first place, no one got pregnant there unless they were thirty-seven. I was only twenty-five. . . . I don't think anyone had ever used their maternity policy. In fact, I don't think they even knew what it was."

Was she bothered? Of course not. "There I was. Pregnant. Perfectly fine. Never sick. Never tired. Never late. Always, 'No guys, I'm fine.' " Her pregnancy passed without a hitch, and to cap off her perfect performance as a liberated woman, she planned to auction off a celebrity's autobiography on her last day of work (the day before her due date). It was to be "a very big deal."

Wakened at four that very morning by labor pains, she did not think, "Oh, maybe I'll have my baby today," but rather, "Oh shit. Can't it just wait?" Much to her husband's dismay, her obstetrician told her there was no reason why she couldn't go to work. "So me and my Lamaze bag and pillow go to the office," she said. There she confided in her secretary and assistant and then pledged them to secrecy. How they managed to maintain it defies imagination. "I swear they never left me. I went to the bathroom, they followed me. I went to Woolworth's to buy slippers . . . they followed me."

She refused calls from her husband, who was being a pest. She auctioned the book; she went out to lunch. "I was in labor, but I totally, mentally distracted myself." At five o'clock, Lamaze bag discreetly hidden, she went downstairs to check out with her boss. He leaned back in his chair and together they reminisced about the success of the auction. Then, rousing himself, he said, "Great. Now you can go home, relax, and have your baby."

Even though Carol's perception of birth is considerably more sober now than it was then, she obviously relishes the next moment in her story. "I said, 'You know, Clint, that's exactly what I'm going to do.'" Whereupon "NO! NO!" lurched from Clint's throat. He sprang from his chair and stumbled downstairs to get her a taxi. Quite enjoying her contrapuntal grace, Carol followed him, stepped into the taxi, went home, had some dinner, went to the hospital, and at 12:31 A.M., gave birth to her first child. "It was the perfect corporate birth," she says, all but applauding her coup.

Hannah, who is also in her early thirties, hasn't Carol's sense of humor or play. So deep is her love of her work, though, that liberation would have had to be invented for her had it not already begun. She has degrees from two prestigious institutions and presently holds an upper-level management position in a major international corporation. It was summer when we met her outside the mid-Manhattan skyscraper in which she works. She was wearing a simple cotton dress. Under its short sleeves, we saw shoulder muscles that were not smooth, but small and twiney, as if she used them to live by. She even seemed to smell of basic work, like woodworking, and it was only when she described how she solved problems that one could sense the highly disciplined quality of her mind. Hannah seems to be doing what is, for her, "right" work; it is mere accident that her craft is corporate and her formidable skills mental. Like others who are compelled by an inner vocational certainty—to write or paint or act or build—and who have the chance to do so, she seems humble. She mentioned several times in our conversation how grateful she was to have the opportunity to do her work.

In the mid-eighties, Hannah and her husband began to think seriously about having a child. The attendant problem was job preservation. Applying the analytic skills that must have contributed to her remarkable success, she assessed the pregnancy tolerances in her particular corporate climate. She ran a mental calculation on upper management, sorting for sex (a very small percentage of women were at the top), marriage (implied stability), parenthood (for women, it preceded entry into upper management), number of children (most women, if they had them at all, had one), and career progress. She factored in soft data. On the negative side, "Yes, there are still sexist jokes, yes, there are still men who pinch you in the elevator," but they were disappearing. On the positive side, the president of the corporation had recently opened the boardroom for a birth shower for a middle-management woman. All things considered, she concluded that her pregnancy would fit within the corporate mold. She planned her pregnancy so that it would coincide with the end of a major project.

Making such a careful decision did not free her from anxiety. She was "nervous about telling. I didn't know how it would go over. I did care about that job a lot." She decided not to say anything for the first few months and to her relief "they didn't notice the boxes [of Special K, which she was living on] in my pocket or the bananas. . . . I stopped drinking coffee but no one noticed that. I used to go to my office at lunchtime and close the door and lie down on the couch for an hour and a half, but I tend to take two-hour lunches so no one knew."

Those were factors she could control. What is much more telling, however, about the influence of the workplace on pregnancy is that her body joined her in the bluff. Although she was very nauseous (thus the Special K) she never threw up at work. "It wasn't discipline," she said. "I don't know what it was. . . . My body knew." Seeming to sense the tightrope she was walking, it reserved its retching demands for off hours. "I'd throw up once or twice during the week [at night] and on weekends, I'd make up for it with a vengeance."

As it turned out, Hannah's anxiety about jeopardizing her position in the company was unnecessary. While she was on maternity leave, they gave her her first set of stock options. "There aren't a lot of people who get them . . . and I was one and that made me feel good." After she returned to work, they provided her with a home computer.

The corporation's acceptance of her pregnancy leads Hannah to conclude that progress has been made on the woman's front. She feels sure that a woman in her position in the mid-seventies would have been thought to have been "not interested in the company" had she gotten pregnant. But while the prejudice seems to have eroded— just because one is pregnant, one is not, therefore, disinterested—the criteria for performance remain the same. Women have broken the bias against the pregnant women not because the business world has accepted, in a generous fashion, the requirements of reproduction, but because women like Hannah and Carol fashioned their reproductive activities to fit the corporate model. Thus, Hannah is thrilled—her face floods with light when she speaks of her child—by her daughter's growth, not from day to day but from weekend to weekend.

Hannah and Carol are exceptional women. Furthermore, they both worked, at the time of their first pregnancies, in exceptionally competitive settings. The influences on them during those pregnancies, however, are not unlike those most women, working for satisfaction or necessity, face during their pregnancies. Work, pregnancy, and birth do not comfortably mesh. As a culture, in fact, we are just beginning—witness the slow acceptance of the need for child care—to admit that childbearing and rearing do influence our lives. In the meantime, women are experiencing their pregnancies in a climate not of motherhood but of separation from it.

The Liberated Birth

The feminist movement has taught women to be in control. In control of destiny, job, financial interests, intellectual and creative life, reproductive self, and daily schedule. A marketing professional commented, "At work, it's mastering and controlling and making things happen when and how you want them to happen." A lawyer called her life "perfect" precisely because it went according to plan. "My life has always been perfect. I planned to go to college. I planned to practice law. I planned to have my child. Everything was perfect." A tax administrator pregnant with her first child remarked, "I like to control everything," and said she would have preferred to plan what her baby was going to look like, what its personality would be, and when it would come.

Liberated, succeeding women have cesarean sections more com-

monly than do other women. "Educated and professional women
. . . are more likely to have cesarean surgery than most other
women,"[3] one study reports, certifying the anecdotal reports we
heard from educated and professional women themselves. This in
spite of the fact that such women generally enjoy better health than
the population at large and that they can afford prenatal care and
specialized medicine.

The situation, which defies medical explanation, invites a holistic
one. Women birth as they live, we recall. If that is so, then succeeding
women will attempt to be in control at birth and, birth, having its
own plans, will sabotage them.

The body-directed birth is gutsy and organic; it does not respect
structure, linear planning, or bottom lines. One woman said birth
was a "freak" event. Another woman, pulling her nostrils up in
disgust, described it as "primitive." "To those of us who live in
cities," a New York City literary agent remarked, birth seems to
resemble "slaughtering a pig."

Natural birth threatens mastery over self and environment. It is
anarchistic. Labor triggers itself without reference to schedule and
can spurt its amniotic fluid out onto a corporate carpet. It doesn't
respect the "birth plans" a conscientious woman is told to draw up.
It's not just emergencies, which are exceptional, but all the bulging,
oozing effects: sweat, pee, and defecation. One may feel one's body
heaving or hear one's throat making primitive, guttural sounds. One
might be mesmerized by hormones and drift off to some altered state.
One may yearn to be held, comforted, and taken care of. At the very
least, one must depend on others to guard one's margins. One is, by
definition, vulnerable.

For the woman whose opportunities in life are dependent on her
freedom from her reproductive rhythms, the roiling animal nature of
the undisturbed birth is threatening. For the woman whose success
derives from her ability to plan and control, its untamable force may
be unacceptable. For the woman who has learned to depend largely
on herself, the prospect of leaning on others may well be terrifying.

The manifesto of the liberated woman is control, which is said to
be the source of her freedom and success. The woman, the feminists
taught, loses everything if she loses control.

In Search of the Liberated Birth

In preliberation days, women learned haphazardly about "what would happen to them" in the hospital from the stories their friends told. One prepared for birth, not by exercising or practicing breathing, but by attending Red Cross Baby Care classes that ignored birth itself. The clear implication was that doctor would do the birth and mother would take up afterward.

With liberation, women set out to reclaim control over their lives and their bodies. In 1969 in Boston a group of women attended a woman's conference, "one of the first gatherings of women meeting specifically to talk with other women." Out of that encounter, smaller groups continued the exploration. One set of women calling themselves the "doctors group" discovered that they shared feelings about doctors, whom they described as being "condescending, paternalistic, judgmental and non-informative." The male physician, who had been at liberty to broadcast his stupefying drugs, to do whatever he liked in the delivery room, was an obvious problem for women seeking self-respect.

Working together on the papers that were to become *Our Bodies, Our Selves,* however, the women's understanding of the problem broadened, and with it their mission. Among other things, they observed that many of their number had not only been "nudged . . . into a fairly rigid role of wife-and-motherhood," but that "many of us were still getting pregnant when we didn't want to." The book that evolved out of their discussions, therefore, was less a criticism of doctors (although that was there) than a device for strengthening women. As, for example, when they researched the fundamentals of conceptual planning and translated them into language any woman could understand. With knowledge on her side, a woman might not have to find herself "playing the role of mother if it is not a role that fits us." Being able to control conception, she might have "a sense of a larger life space to work in, an invigorating and challenging sense of time and room to discover the energies and talents that are in us, to do the work we want to do."[4]

For good reason, the book became a landmark publication for feminists. Not only did it cover the territory, not only did it have scope, perspicacity, and intelligence, but it had a disarming style. Reading it, one felt at home at last with a book about one's body. One was not instructed, but joined. Effortlessly, it seemed, the authors of *Our Bodies, Our Selves* found a quiet voice of self-respect—usually so shifty—and held it. We had permission to care, intelligently and nondefensively, about our female health.

Interested as they were in providing women with the knowledge they need to plan their childbearing, the authors were equally interested in the quality of birth. The woman who freely chooses to have a child, who learns about her body and emotions during pregnancy and prepares herself for the birth experience, may be rewarded by "full excitement and joy," an experience enlarged by the feeling of connectedness it invites. "As women giving birth, we are connected through time and space to all other women who have ever given birth. Rather than being ordinary, it is a profound experience, worthy of respect. That the process of labor and delivery is universal to all mothers, everywhere and at all times, dignifies our experience even further."[5]

The way to obtain a quality experience was to gain control. "Most important, by preparing ourselves for childbirth we will be giving ourselves more control over our experience."[6] By educating one's mind and body, by taking back the responsibility for making decisions about one's body, women could direct their births and have the physicians and hospitals working for them, rather than the other way around.

Nature's Control

Regaining control meant, inevitably, tackling afresh the problem of pain in childbirth. Pain, after all, had provoked women to choose scopolamine and, because of it, they had submitted to the will of their physicians. The authors of *Our Bodies, Our Selves,* researching alternatives for relief of pain in labor, mentioned two seminal works in childbirth education, both of which offered methods by which women could reinvolve themselves in the birth process.

Grantly Dick-Read's book, *Childbirth Without Fear,* argued

that birth pain was caused by fear. Fear restricted blood circulation in the uterus; restricted blood circulation gave rise to pain; therefore, the frightened uterus was a painful uterus. With a boldness that seemed to amaze even him, Dick-Read proclaimed that pain was unnecessary. He told how he attended the birth of a young woman who completed her birth efficiently at home and said afterward, "It wasn't meant to [hurt] was it, doctor?" Women who were not predisposed to fear birth, he theorized, did not experience pain. The idea that they had to was myth, a distortion of civilization. To prove his point, he went so far as to uncover scholarly evidence showing that the Bible, where it said that women should give birth in pain, had been mistranslated. The original Hebrew, correctly read, said that women birthed not in pain but in labor, as one labors in the fields. Pain was not dictated by women's birthing bodies but by civilization, which conditioned women to be frightened of birth.

Dick-Read's childbirth education method, therefore, was designed to teach women to untie the tight civilized knots they were heir to. If a woman was confident and relaxed during birth, he observed, she naturally labored herself into a state (resembling the one Odent describes) that was "carefree," "semi-conscious," and "amnesic." With it came surcease of pain. "As the level of consciousness is lowered still further, so the sensations of labor cease to be painful."[7] If a woman knew enough about birth, therefore, she could eradicate civilization's misteachings and relinquish her body to its more natural laboring state. By exercising, practicing relaxation, and learning some breathing techniques, he said she could birth painlessly.

For all his faith in the laboring woman's body, Dick-Read did not believe a woman should give birth in animallike isolation. Humans enjoy society. Drawing from his battlefield experiences in World War I, he argued that pain was influenced by outward circumstances and other people. Pain felt more unbearable when one was alone and frightened, as he had been one interminable night tending the wounded and dying of Gallipoli, explosions shattering the perimeters of the universe, and he with no one to make the simplest exchange. He only wanted someone to whom he could say, "What do you think happened?" Being alone, the healthy healer grew shaky, light of head, and by morning was ashen faced.

Pain increased when a person was tired, weary of mind, and depressed. A person who felt alone would think of nothing but pain. The caregiver who wanted to help a woman to sink into painlessness, therefore, would create an environment of peace and comfort. The caregiver needed to be patient, quiet, understanding, honest, gentle, peaceful, confident, interested, cheerful, and attentive and so communicate to the woman that all was well. Then she would birth "undisturbed and confident."

The 1930s medical establishment, absorbed in solving the problems of modern women and hospital birth, was not impressed by Dick-Read's book. Joseph DeLee was of the opinion that "it would take seven thousand generations before we can train women back to the state which Grantly Dick-Read speaks of in 'Natural Childbirth.' "[8] Fernand Lamaze, who followed Dick-Read as a major figure in childbirth education, observed: "Needless to say, his theories met with strong opposition from both the British medical world and the Anglican Church and resulted in Dick-Read being shunned, if not abused."[9] Like midwives, Dick-Read was not appreciated for his interest in nature's way.

Intellectual Control

Lamaze, a Frenchman, admired Dick-Read, but thought that his neurophysiology was flawed. The proof was right there in his results, which showed that women who used his methods did *not* regularly lapse into the painless and mystical state that Dick-Read described. No, Lamaze argued, the pain pathways of the human animal were not the same as those of unthinking creatures; furthermore, a human was more than a physical being and "this doctrine of natural childbirth is fast becoming a simple matter of muscle activity, like some stupid athletic performance."[10]

He, by contrast, recommended that a woman employ her higher intelligence to avoid pain: "a brain that organizes the activities of the body and is always in touch with the functions of its organs." There-

fore it could be retrained, "and the influence of consciousness . . .
teaches a woman to deliver herself without pain."[11] By learning to
barricade some of her nerve corridors, by siderailing the painful
messages, a woman could avoid, not having pain, but perceiving it.

While the burden of the responsibility for short-circuiting pain
was on the conscious woman, her caregivers, like Dick-Read's, were
to abet her. The birthplace should grant her privacy and low lights.
Birth attendants should be gentle, kind, understanding, calm, and
knowledgeable. "Every woman who walks into the Maternity Unit
must feel she is surrounded by friends who are eager to bear with her
and help her."[12] Women should be nourished, tended, and supported
not for sentimental reasons, but so pain would be less.

Although Lamaze's book, *Painless Childbirth,* was not published
in America until 1970, his ideas were popularized here by Marjorie
Karmel's 1959 book, *Thank You, Dr. Lamaze.* Living in France
during her first pregnancy, Karmel had studied with a Lamaze childbirth educator. That woman had instructed her, "You must not
think of it as taking it easy. That would be too passive." Taking it
easy, letting go, becoming passive, would "only slow down the activity of your brain, which in turn . . . would increase your sensitivity
to pain."[13]

For women who were determined, once and for all, to take control
over their lives and their bodies, for women infuriated by the price
passive women had paid in childbirth, the Lamaze method had
obvious attractions. For one thing, according to the American Society for Prophylaxis in Obstetrics (ASPO), the organization formed
to promote the Lamaze method in the States, it was decidedly not
natural: "It is wholly artificial, a completely contrived and man-
made way of dealing with uterine contractions in labor."[14] Thus
women finding their liberation need not fear falling back into the
grasp of the "possessive," "preying" nature that de Beauvoir had first
warned them of. Quite to the contrary, the Lamaze method fit well
with their urge to employ their freshly reclaimed minds and redis-
covered wills.

Making it all the more attractive to the American woman, who
was flushed with principles of self-determination, the Lamaze
method, as interpreted by its New World advocates, implied that she

needed little help from others to succeed. In making the transatlantic crossing, Lamaze's privacy, low lights, gentle, kind, and attentive caregivers, etc., were left behind. The ASPO nearly ignored environmental factors in their book *Awake and Aware.* Like a frontiersman, a woman was to rely almost entirely on her own resources. For support, which she should not expect from hospital staff (or so it is vaguely implied), she would depend upon her Lamaze-trained husband, whose responsibility was to be an informed presence and to "act as a sort of coach, timing contractions and keeping the woman doing the techniques properly."[15]

We must note, not so tangentially, what an untenable position this put her husband in. He was a relative newcomer to female anatomy and physiology. He was ignorant but for a few classes about birth. He was a nobody in the hospital institution. He was becoming a father. And yet we asked him to be the "coach" of his wife's body during her labor. We asked him to witness her pain and beat off those unscrupulous intervenors who offered to dull it. We asked him to establish the drumbeat of her breathing. We asked him, in some ways, to be even more in control, more distanced, than she.

We wonder why men can't be emotionally looser. We complain that they don't feel more and manage less. But for all those years that Lamaze was in vogue, we asked them to maintain high discipline during one of the most powerful emotional passages in life. It indicates how completely we lost our bearings. We asked men to become feeling fathers, but we arranged it so that they had, above all, to remain managers. We did the same to women.

Armed Control

In 1972, Capitol Records released Helen Reddy's recording of "I Am Woman." Its call-to-courage lyrics praised women's wisdom, which was, apropos of our subject, "born of pain," and they urged her to expunge forever the indignities she had suffered. Helen Reddy belted, "I am strong/I am invincible/I am woman," and the women who listened to her song were the same ones who learned that they were to give birth in defiance of the medical establishment.

In the 1976 edition of *Our Bodies, Our Selves,* with heat *and* light, the authors reported doctors' pathological view of birth and the hospitals' inhospitality toward the wholeness of woman. They said that the woman who appreciated her dignity as childbearer would be up against formidable obstacles when she entered the hospital. They also implied that she could manage.

It was a poignant moment in the history of women at birth. The authors understood that institutions victimized women. They also understood that the hospitals would continue to victimize women until the women challenged them. Therefore the women, drawing on an embryonic sense of their worth as females, had to prepare themselves not only to control pain and birth, but to do both in a brightly lighted, nonprivate, ungentle, impatient, and often hostile environment.

This birth strategy, presented with the same serenity and sureness that pervades *Our Bodies, Our Selves,* is half defense and half offense. The woman was to prepare herself for birth by learning about reproduction, by practicing Lamaze breathing and concentration methods, and by finding a birth companion who would support and protect her on her journey. Once in labor, she was to report to a hospital, where she would receive, as welcome, a shave and enema. With those procedures accomplished, she was to advise her caregivers that she intended to be "actively involved" in her labor from start to finish. Forthwith, she would begin to monitor their activities, to be sure that they checked her vital signs at appropriate intervals. As her labor progressed she was to measure its development against her knowledge of the normal progress of labor, and if she discovered some deviance, she would "keep complaining until someone listens to you." During transition, she was not only to "be careful" about the temptation she might feel to take drugs, but also to insist that a nurse remain by her side until the phase passed. Then, in defiance of virtually all hospital policy at that time (and revealing the influence of midwifery on the authors), she was to squat, semisquat or side-lie and push out her baby.[16]

In other words, she was to dominate, during her "great emergency," not only her body but the entire institutional order of American birth.

Imposition of Reality

"It is not unusual for Lamaze prepared women in the United States to receive some narcotic analgesia or even epidural anesthesia during labor," *Williams Obstetrics* advises. Certainly, among the women we talked to, it was not unusual. One woman arrived at the hospital, a few hours of labor behind her, the baby's head swelling her perineum, and ordered, "Put in some medicine, fast!" "I was not, am not ideologically opposed to taking something," said another. One more mentioned, without comment or interest, that she received Seconal during the first slow stages of her labor and later Demerol. "I would have liked an epidural but it went too fast," she added. "I hate to put birth on the level of dentistry," another said, "[but I asked myself] would I have a tooth pulled without anything?" An editor, preparing for a drug-free birth with a midwife, was surrounded by her friends at the shower they gave her. "Take drugs," they urged, taking her aside one by one. "Take drugs."

Many mocked the idea that a woman should endure pain—they classified it as machisma. Why bother, as Leslie in the first chapter said, "for the sake of some ideal." Another said, "I didn't see any reason to be brave. . . . I think you can be ridiculous about going through all this pain for what? To say that you've gone through natural childbirth?" We found the most dramatic statement of the antisuffering attitude in an angry article for *Parenting* magazine: "When friends assured me that I could 'take it [the drugless birth],' I countered by asking, 'Why should I?' After all, Americans on the whole embrace the notion of pain relief—our burgeoning over-the-counter and prescription drug market attests to that. . . . Childbirth, I pointed out, involved severe, prolonged pain."[17]

Among these succeeding women, the fulfilling birth described in *Our Bodies, Our Selves* seems to have gone the way of sandals and beads. The serene woman, master of her pain and environment, has vanished. In her place comes a woman who is assertive about being pacified at birth. Today's breed of woman, many observers complain, can't be bothered with discomfort: It's "me, me, me," they are accused of saying. Others note that women will often present that attitude mid-pregnancy, but as they become more attached to the child in later pregnancy, they change and want only what's best for their baby. Then they are accused of contributing to the interventionist practices in medicine because they demand a "perfect birth" and a "perfect child." "They," the women, "want the ultrasounds" to make sure everything is perfect; "they" want the amniocentecis, the AFP, and nonstress tests to prove that the child is faultless; "they" write a birth plan; "they" want to maintain their composure during birth; "they" ask for the perfectly balanced, precisely administered drugs; "they" are the ones upon whom you'd better put a fetal monitor because if the baby's not perfect, they'll sue.

And yet somewhere in these women's minds (and we talked to many very bright, well-educated women) is the information that drugs cross into the baby's bloodstream; that epidurals suppress their central nervous system and those of their babies; that the chance of a forceps delivery is increased by three to five times when there's been an epidural; and that you can't get up and move about when you're on a fetal monitor, which can further suppress the baby's vitality, which may cause a drop in the fetal heartbeat and prompt a cesarean.

These are perfect births? Ones that end up with forceps and c-sections? These are the methods that informed, intelligent women employ to produce the most responsive, brightest, cleverest child, the most "perfect" child?

Prepared Childbirth

It is now believed that Lamaze, like Dick-Read before him, made some mistakes. In fact, some of his critics say, his ideas were "a step backward." All he did, they say, was to substitute one kind of control—the kind the anesthetic-carrying doctor could provide—with another, which the self-armed woman would self-induce. Furthermore, the pure Lamaze method asked women to internalize the hospital's standards of the good patient: Be orderly and predictable; don't make a disturbance; stay distant from your labor so you can be "in control"; and underneath that—don't get too involved. Lamaze-prepared women conscientiously "houted" and panted and breathed, and their husbands counted and coached. But while some of this attention to breathing seemed to help, the claim of painless childbirth, everyone had to admit, was much overrated.

Other theories have drifted into the mix of advice. Sheila Kitzinger was one who suggested that Lamaze erred in emphasizing control. Birth, she said, was a psychosexual experience and went better if a woman let herself go with it, the way she did with sex. Just as one didn't "achieve" orgasm in intercourse by mentally coercing one's body, one did not give birth by direction, as if it were a flight plan. Kitzinger, notable for being the only mother among the big heads in childbirth education, found the Lamaze and other "psychoprophylactic" methods repressive. They "have tended to emphasize the lack of painful sensations, but have, perhaps to the cost of some of those mothers who have adopted them, neglected that exhilaration which comes in a creative experience of completely harmonious psycho-physical functioning."[18] More in line with Read, Odent, and today's holists, she said that a lively birth—even with its "background" of pain—gave the woman something. It is an experience "through which we grow to greater spiritual and psychological fullness."[19] One did not enjoy these benefits by systematically avoiding the messages coming from one's body, but by listening to them.

In this country, the responsive, participatory birth was recommended by Robert A. Bradley, MD. Like other birth reformers, he theorized that civilization may have distorted women's capacity to give birth, but there was no reason why they couldn't reclaim their animal capacity. "Women can give birth by the action of their own bodies, as animals do. Women can enjoy the process of birth and add to their dignity by being educated to follow the example set by instinctive animals."[20] His techniques, which involve the husband extensively, are similar to those recommended by Kitzinger in that they teach a woman to go with her labor.

Much to the layperson's confusion, all schools of thought—from DeLee's to Odent, from the most technocratically oriented to the most earthy—seem to have the same goal. Do it this way, their exponents write winningly, and you will be *in control.* When doctors and Lamaze-type educators make the claim, it makes some sense; but how do the Kitzinger, Bradley, Odent types—poeticizing about rhythms and yieldings, dare speak of control? And yet Kitzinger promises a "beautifully controlled labor."[21]

It may be helpful to simplify the debate. Essentially, there are two schools of thought. The one endorsed generally by the medical profession and by early Lamaze supporters views birth and nature with suspicion. Their birth devices—whether chemical, technological, or psychological—are meant to grip nature and keep her squirmy, squealy tendencies in one's hand. The other, represented by Read, Kitzinger, Bradley, Odent, and a variety of present-day holists, give nature some credit.

When doctors and Lamaze used the word control, they meant control over nature. One is to dominate the process. In the doctor's use, this translates into popping the amniotic sack, timing labor precisely, measuring contractions religiously, restructuring internal chemistry, applying forceps and scalpels. In the Lamaze translation, precision is equally valued. One thinks of husbands and wives, scrupulously tracking breaths and minutes. The watchwords of Lamaze are "suppression" and "inhibition."

The Kitzinger-Bradley-Odent-holist method recommends control through nature. One attends one's physiological voice; one credits the information coming from one's body and one's psyche; one follows one's impulses. In birth, control is not obtained through conflict but by coordination. Kitzinger, who uses the ripest language, writes: "Bodies are for feeling with, and for actively living through and enjoying. When the healthy human body is engaged in a natural physiological process the individual normally feels pleasure and content: we enjoy eating and drinking and defecating, settling down to sleep and waking refreshed, walking and swimming, breathing the sea air and making love."[22] Birth, she says, can feel as satisfying.

One of the most striking differences between the two schools of thought is that one promises only absence of pain and a bottom-line product, a baby. Technologically oriented doctors, for example, speak of getting their patients "through"; and one can search Lamaze for some mention of human growth, love for the child, some indication of a larger experience and find only anatomy, physiology, personal hygiene, and exercises.

The other crowd, which also promise a baby at the end, tend to fulminate with expressions of meaning, liveliness, insight, and love.

Dick-Read gives us "beauty," and "exhilaration and intense joy." After a good birth, Kitzinger says, a woman "experiences the glow of health and well-being and an overwhelming joy. She may feel that she has been enabled to share in the work of creation." She and her husband "have experienced together something incomprehensibly wonderful—a peak of joy in their married life which will perhaps always be for them a symbol of the deepest sort of love they know."[23] Bradley quotes clients who say that birth was the "most beautiful experience of my life," and observes, "After twenty-six years and well over thirteen thousand attended births by natural childbirth I have often stated that the only handicap I have found in the method is the superenthusiasm of the parents afterward. They will talk your arm off."[24]

Odent, immaculately, makes no attempt to describe what it feels like to be a woman and give birth, but he does reveal his enthusiasm for pregnancy and birth. Writing about his weekly sings for pregnant and postpartum mothers at Pithiviers, he says, "It is a pleasure to sing and dance. And pleasure must not be underrated; it can only enhance pregnancy."[25] He quotes the women: "Eddie lowers me and they put the baby in my arms. I am stunned: not a word is spoken. The baby cries a bit and starts looking for the nipple. All is so peaceful and so intense." He also gives us a midwife's expression of the fullness of the birth moment.

> I am overcome. There is nothing to teach her. She pushes for life on her own. I am not to touch her. . . . She is creative, inventive, full of life. She looks for what she wants. She is exhausted and yet so vital. As she throws herself upon me, I am covered in her sweat. I am obliged to do as she wishes. But she is beautiful, she is the life that she is about to bring forth. She no longer asks me the time, the sex, the weight. Instead, she simply cries out with pleasure.[26]

Odent himself exults quietly: "Though we have watched this scene thousands of times, we still look on with endless wonder."

Very few of the women we talked with mentioned wonder. They recounted stoical ordeals; something necessary, hard and not especially rewarding in and of itself. Hannah had "some pain stuff" and some time later, they "took me out of the birthing room and rolled me into the labor room and used forceps to pull her [the baby] out." Another woman "got her baby." The lawyer who held her arm out for drugs "delivered" her child. The one who accepted the Seconal and Demerol "was torn up pretty far inside." For a highly Lamaze-prepared woman—her husband had a stopwatch—"the delivery was accomplished."

Those who were affected had somehow been overtaken by the process: Carol, the woman who managed that "perfect corporate birth," recalled that the urge to push overwhelmed her: "It was the most incredible moment of being totally out of control . . . I couldn't have stopped it . . . I was kind of amazed. . . . Astounding." Another woman who delivered drug-free (not on purpose) said: "The experience was so nice . . . it was so intimate, close. . . . My husband kissed me and I think I will always have a nice, warm, wonderful, content feeling from that birth. It was just special." Another woman, a recovering alcoholic, was very anxious to have a drug-free birth. At the crucial moment (just before birth) she, like so many women, lost heart and asked her midwife for something. The midwife asked her if she could just hold on a little longer and "I found the pain sort of glorious."

And finally: "I experienced a kind of transcendent state. I felt like I was no longer chained to my body or even a part of it. I was just watching. As I looked in the mirror it was as if my baby was coming to me from the heavens. I saw his body unfold toward me . . . I wasn't tired anymore, just in awe."

The Sting

Hᴀʀᴅʟʏ ᴀɴʏᴏɴᴇ anymore will say that there isn't pain with childbirth; but childbirth educators, we also understand, speak little of the emotional rewards that may accrue to the mother who surrenders to birth. Instead, many of them rigorously follow the International Childbirth Education Association (ICEA) motto: Informed choice through the knowledge of alternatives. Respecting a woman's right to choose, they present her with choices. In this, of course, they are limited by what is available.

Pennsylvania Hospital is a choice in Philadelphia, for example. Although they have recently opened that midwife-run Birthing Suite,[1] the majority of births still take place on a traditional labor and delivery floor. Those who give the tours and explain the policies are quick to point out, up front, that theirs is a higher-tech unit than most because they are a tertiary care center, i.e., prepared for especially high-risk cases. Nevertheless, they do their share of what are called "normal births."

To the left, as one enters the unit, are cubbyholes, each one equipped with a bed and a fetal monitor. The laboring woman, we are told, will position herself on one of the beds in order to have a sample "strip" taken on the fetal monitor. It establishes that she is indeed in labor and also provides a base for later comparisons. Her vagina is inspected with a speculum (a metal instrument) and her vital signs are measured and recorded. Those women who have had babies before and have no apparent complications are assigned to labor rooms to the front of the unit; the others are referred to the back of the unit to be nearer the delivery and operating rooms.

To get to their rooms women pass by the nurses' station. It's a long, low, white module which, with its computer screen overhead, provokes thoughts of space launchings. Behind the desk is a bank of glass-faced shelves stacked with boxes of needles, syringes, exam gloves, and the like. A phone installation spreads across the center of the desk and its buttons buzz and flash.

Someone in white fills out a stack of charts. A beeper sounds. Somebody else picks up the phone, calls her husband, and asks him to bring her her glasses, which she forgot; another person puzzles aloud over what to have for lunch. "Where's that c-sec?" a nurse inquires. "She's in five," another answers. "Would you check three and four for me?" the first one says.

A nondescript woman enters the labor and delivery unit. A vacant look on her face, she stands in the corridor near the nurses' station, clutching her purse. After a few minutes, she is spoken to. We overhear that she's in premature labor. She sits down in a straight-backed chair near the door to the unit and stares at the floor. A young, tall, dark-haired doctor wanders past her to the nurses' station, chats for a few minutes, strolls over to the cabinet, picks up an Amni-hook, absentmindedly slaps it against his palm. "I think I want to rupture her membranes," he says, referring to one of his patients, and he wanders over to a room marked by a brown sign impressed with white lettering. "Patient," it reads.

From behind the nurses' station one can see directly into four of these labor rooms. Each is about as wide as a subway car and about a third as long. The walls are green and illuminated by flourescent light. Cramped up next to the bed is a stainless steel trolley and a confusion of equipment. We're told that the noncomplicated woman who labors in these rooms may have three to five attachments made to her. She will have a "lock" put in her arm, which means she can be given fluids, drugs, and blood intravenously, having only to be punctured once. There's the datascope for the epidural, the belts for the fetal monitor, the Pitocin on a pump, and possibly oxygen. If she's uncomfortable and not on continuous monitoring, she can get up and walk around. At the moment, no one is taking advantage of this opportunity.

Kitty-corner to the head of the bed is one of those secretary's chairs with the short back, the metal base, and wheels. Although it is meant for him, the husband generally does not use the chair. He stands by his wife's head, which is remarkable considering the amount of space left for him there. A small table is positioned just outside the door. At it sits a woman in white. She has a clipboard and appears to be tracking the events that occur inside the room.

The doctor with the Amni-hook enters one of the laboring rooms and shuts the door. A few minutes later he emerges. He walks past the woman in premature labor, still sitting there, her purse clutched to her belly.

> Every woman who walks into the Maternity Unit must feel she is surrounded by friends who are eager to be with her and help her.[2]

Riding on a metal gurney, a woman near delivery breaks through swinging doors and into a corridor banked on either side by carts heaped with green sheets and stacked with stainless steel receptacles. Passing through another swinging door, she rides onto the delivery room floor, which is black and nubby, like a parking lot. To her left, nearly wall to wall, ceiling to floor, are metal drawers and cabinets. To her right, tables, warming lights, an isolette, instruments wrapped in packs. Blocking a window is a metal installation. It has tubes hanging from it, a bellows in a jar, buttons, switches, cords. A vast mirror and huge orange lights, like satellites, loom over the delivery table.

A woman who trusts her body and who feels safe can relax. Relaxation lets her labor go. It lets the body's natural pain-killers flood. In a darkened, quiet, protected space, with companions who are warm and supportive, she will labor effectively and her pain—that "background"—will be suffused with a feeling of rightness, naturalness and power.

St. Joseph's Hospital in Lancaster, Pennsylvania, advertises their birthing rooms in the local newspaper. We take the elevator to the fifth floor to see it. The doors swish open and we are swamped in a purplish light. We must be either orchids in a hothouse or aliens, landed in a sci-fi laboratory on another planet. And so we rush past the bilirubin-lighted baby nursery. The hospital's childbirth educator greets us and leads us to the birthing rooms. She pushes the heavy, wheelchair-wide door open, and we enter a huge room decorated with curtained windows, flowered bedspread, oval mirror, rocking chair. The bed, she says, after we admire the decor, "breaks down." "Why is that?" "There are doctors here who prefer to have the women on their backs when they deliver. Some of them don't know how to do side-lying deliveries."

"And why is the room so big?" we ask.

Our guide leads us around the corner, sheepishly opens a closet, and out of it peers, like eyes in the night, a virtual army of obstetrical robots. They toe the closet's threshold. "Is there room for the husband after these roll into the room?" we ask. "He tends to step out of the way," she says.

Birth goes best when a woman can believe in her body and lose herself in intimacy.

At Dartmouth-Hitchcock Hospital, on their own time, the nurses redecorated the old labor rooms. They hung wallpaper, had matching curtains made up, and found rocking chairs. In the hallways, in the delivery room, they stood on ladders and patiently stenciled a country border print onto the walls. It is a place, said Anne-Marie Disco, a labor and delivery nurse, "where people really do get excited about a normal birth."

We stood in the small room. There were some electronic tendrils creeping out of the wallpaper, a formica-topped tray table crowded the corner, a bulletlike television set projected from the wall, but still, the room was inviting—like a bedroom in a bed and breakfast. Since working at Hitchcock, Anne-Marie has come to believe that tension does inhibit a woman's birth. On the other hand, she said, sometimes "people come together for a birth" and everything flows together. They work shoulder to shoulder, their bodies and their minds blend, their needs transmit without words—not just caregiver to client, but caregiver to caregiver—and sometimes, in those instances, birth surpasses itself and it feels spiritual.

And then, breaking off, she demonstrated how the back of the birthing bed could be cranked up to support the woman's back (which precludes a human hold) and how a metal rod could be raised by her side (which bars a human hand). As we left the room, Anne-Marie said it would be amusing to know which television programs were on most during births.

An English childbirth educator said that women seem to search for their mothers when they anticipate labor. They yearn for lap, plump arms, flannely wrap, and loving face. They know instinctively, perhaps, that they must be free to lose themselves in their bodies and depend on others, as infants must, to protect them with their hearts and minds while they do. These women today, torn from their mothers at birth and for some days afterward, may beat away the desire.

The childbirth educator who talks to these women often finds herself between a rock and a hard place. If she understands that birth can be repressed by tension, disruption, and a climate of distrust, what does she say to her students, most of whom will be having their babies under a doctor's care and in a hospital? To commend them to natural childbirth is almost cruel. If natural birth is a function of warmth and embrace and if hospitals are cool and mechanical, then how perverse it is to say: Succeed.

Doctors say to their patients, "You can try for natural childbirth. Go as far as you can and then if you want something, we'll give it to you." "We hope," childbirth educators say to their students, "that you will make it, but you mustn't feel guilty if you don't." "Informed choice," says the ICEA, "based on knowledge of the alternatives." Women who give birth in hospitals, Michel Odent says, probably do need pain relief medication.

Double Bind

We do not woo women into giving birth. We do not trail our fingertips on the beds we've made up, anticipating their coming. We do not bake their favorite bread, pick flowers, hurry down the path to greet them, settle down with them, and ask them about their trip. We do not suggest that they make themselves at home. We do not say, "What can I get you?" We do not touch them, rejoice in them, admire them, laugh with them, or stand by them. We do not treat them as if they were all our daughters, whom we have adored and who are taking up major work. For some reason, we have chosen to show little love.

As if warmth and hospitality were bad things, we distance ourselves and treat birthing women like strangers who have booked a room in a motel. We expect them to manage on their own and often humiliate them if they don't. We ask them to be independent and in control. We surround them with machinery. Too often we provide only peremptory, distant, and objective care. We tell them the rules they must follow. We measure their body's performance and pronounce it adequate or inadequate (Lamaze attempted/Lamaze failed), as if they were in a competition. We make birth a cold test of character and physical performance. It is no wonder women fear birth and are anxious about motherhood, both of which, apparently, must be undertaken alone and in defiance of culture.

We communicate a similar message to babies, whom we drug for the passage into life and yank out with forceps. Whom we needle and stick in plastic boxes, depriving them of the softness of breast and belly. We introduce them to the world harshly, as if to say, "Life's a bastard. All edges and assaults."

How strange it is that those who believe birth is about love and kindness and dignity and caring find themselves on the outside, demanding to be heard. How incomprehensible that they are called radicals and reformers. How absurd that they must gear up, get organized, make speeches, raise money, lobby, and negotiate in order to get others to notice that birth and motherhood have a human dimension.

Childbirth educators do the best they can. They place caring high on their list of their priorities. You can hear it at their conventions— they are outraged by insensitive caregivers and, brows knitted, they devise strategies to make the system more sensitive and responsive. They debate the methods they have for helping pregnant women find the courage to speak for their needs. But in private conversations, they wonder if women will ever be able to speak up. They say they've been too oppressed. Furthermore, they have reason to suspect there will be reprisals for the woman who challenges the system.

Determined to be heard, responding to criticisms that they have been too kitsch to count, childbirth educators have professionalized their message. They have abstracted it into psychologically approved principles. One attempts to reform women and the system by accepting a person "where she is." Above all, the childbirth educator defers to the mother and father to be. She refuses to dictate. She will not ram her opinions or her life experience down her students' throats. She listens, she tries to understand, she answers questions and does her best to honor others' values.

Thus the 1987 "Competencies and Program Guidelines for Nurse Providers of Childbirth Education," which is put out by the Nurses Association of the American College of Obstetricians and Gynecologists (NAACOG), requires its nurse-educators to conduct "consumer needs assessments," to select teaching strategies "suited to the specific group," to foster "independence in learning," and to appreciate "others' values systems." In that context, the nurse disseminates "accurate, scientific, and practical information," as if it were value-free.[3]

The ICEA, whose roots are outside the medical establishment, do not pretend to such lack of bias. They have an opinion on women and birth: They're after "wellness, health promotion, risk reduction, self-involvement, informed consent, birth as a unique experience and use of nonmedical and self-care techniques for normal pregnancy, labor and birth." One might think, therefore, that the woman who plans on being "drugged to the hilt" would be uncomfortable with an ICEA educator.

But, no. "The ultimate choice for care resides with the individual," the ICEA says. The information—such as, the benefits of the self-involvement in birth—is to be given but, like the nurse educators, the ICEA educator must keep her personal values out of the way and let the woman choose. The operative oath is "informed consent."[4]

Margery Simchack, RN, for example, led two long workshops at a 1987 ICEA convention, both of which were concerned with epidural anesthesia. Although she presented with clinical crispness, her material was a willies-making barrage. She threw slides on the screen so we could see how precise the anesthesiologist had to be in placing the point of his needle; otherwise it would stick a hole in the spinal cord. She listed nausea and dizziness as side effects of epidurals. She passed the long, thin, wagging needle around. But just as we were beginning to feel the urge to march on the pharmaceutical companies that manufacture epidural anesthesia, she sternly reminded us: "Remember, there is no such thing as a wrong decision."

The realists in childbirth education understand that information, as cool as it appears to be, is not value-free. If nothing else, the instructor chooses what to present. She has maybe sixteen hours with her students, and within that time there's an ample amount of designated information to be disseminated. One is obliged to cover the parents' emotional and psychological "tasks"; she must provide a cursory explanation of the anatomy and physiology of pregnancy; she will mention sexual adjustments; she is to discuss the common problems of hemorrhoids, bleeding, leaking, cramping, vomiting, vaginal discharges, swelling, varicosities, etc.; she will present information about prenatal screening tests—not just amniocentesis, alphafetoprotein, and ultrasound—but also chorionic villi sampling, nuclear magnetic resonance, and others. Then there's chemical exposure, sexually transmitted diseases, use of alcohol, tobacco, and caffeine, not to mention nutrition and exercise. Finally, she must talk about the hospital and the fetal monitor and the drugs and the surgical procedures. A woman must be prepared to make her choices.

Within this context, of course, the childbirth educator chooses what to emphasize and how to present. Nurses who teach in hospitals, for example, "subconsciously know what these people are going to get," said May Shumaker, an independent childbirth educator from Massachusetts. They can't avoid teaching: "This is what you should know because this is what is going to happen to you." If a nurse-educator knows that the epidural rate in her hospital is 90 percent, she is conscience-bound to prepare her clients for one. If she is employed by a doctor who has a 25 percent cesarean rate, she is unlikely to emphasize how long it takes to recover from major surgery. If she has never seen a natural birth, she will be inclined to say disbelievingly, "Well, you can try."

The "information" one gets from a childbirth educator is chosen, and the way it is chosen is not, for all the piety surrounding the stance, value-free. Neither is its expression value-free. If, for example, an educator has her students practice their breathing while lying flat on their backs, she implies that one labors flat on one's back. If she decides not to show films of women laboring nude (because it's said to make couples uncomfortable), she implies that birth should be covered up. If she says enough times, "We *hope* you will not have any complications," she eventually communicates hopelessness.

The Limits of Subversion

One nurse, leading a tour through a labor ward, advised her group that the hospital recommended that they not eat once they were in labor. "But I had bacon and eggs," she said, subversively. One childbirth educator said she advises her students to "just say No when they say they want to put an IV lock in your arm." Most of the reform-minded try to get their clients in the habit of challenging early on in pregnancy. Beth Shearer, an experienced educator now working with women who are preparing for VBAC, says that it's a matter of getting women to value their own needs. "Parents have a right to medical care which respects their needs," she says. "If you go to a doctor who does 90 percent epidurals . . . it's not fair to expect anything else from him." In that case, she tells women, "It's OK to change providers." The birth plan, used by some educators to help a woman visualize her birth, may be hardened into a negotiating tool. A woman describes how she wants her birth to be conducted and presents it to her physician. If he says, "I don't do that," or, "We'll see how it goes," or "Leave it to me," she's to turn on her heel and find another caregiver.

But a woman during her pregnancy is emotionally labile, they tell us. She's having a healthy, growth crisis that tends to be characterized by introspectiveness and sensitivity. Negotiate, we tell her. Make demands. Defy the medical establishment; defy the representatives of that group of people who have given us in vitro fertilization and in utero surgery. Defy those who are known to save babies. Walk out, you with your ridiculously irrelevant expertise in office management or computer programming or accounting, walk out. You with your uncertainty about your motherhood, about your body, about the changes that are coming in your marriage. Just say no.

Given institutional realities, of course, even the assertive may run into trouble. In some small towns, doctors aren't amenable to accepting patients who went to other doctors first. In cities, in certain HMOs, you take what your designated doctor offers or you have your baby at your own expense. If you're stuck, say the reformers, you still don't need to be a victim. If the doctor puts you on that fetal monitor, if the baby's heartbeat drops, if the people in white start mumbling about a cesarean, then rise. Rise up and walk. Assert your way to the shower. Demand "hugs before drugs."

The trouble with all this, of course, is that it requires superwoman behavior. The trouble with all this, of course, is that it belies the notion that birth works. "Women who come to a childbirth education class don't know anyone who has had a normal birth. Not in the media, in their childhood, in the previous course of pregnancy, in their friends' experience. Nothing reinforces." The trouble with all this, of course, is that it directly contradicts the psychological necessities of birth. "If you are separate enough from your labor to stand free from yourself," Shearer says, "you're too separate to be able to do the labor work." In order to labor well, "You have to give up control to the labor. Go with it."

To solve this problem, we give guard duty to partners. So that she can give up control, he is asked to take it up. We put eight classes on pregnancy and birth under his belt and then, with enormous presumption, we put him in foreign and well-defended territory where he will witness every twitch of his wife's suffering and we ask him to lay down the law. We make it his job to second-guess the nurse's reading of the fetal monitor, to challenge the physician, to say to the anesthesiologist (turning a blind eye to his wife's agonized face), "My wife may say she wants drugs, but she really doesn't want them." He is to push assertively past the crowding machinery and the circling caretakers and demand the right to hold her hand.

It's difficult for man or woman to be a ghetto fighter and an open human being at the same time.

PART V

THE GIVING IN BIRTH

W<small>E HAVE</small> said a number of times that we needn't continue as we have in the birthplace. We have said that there were institutions already up and in operation in which birth did not have to be a fearsome, rigidly controlled event. We said that it is quite possible for ordinary American women to give birth as Amish women do. It seems as if we've had to go a long way in order to get to the point where we can, rather simply, describe the available solution. It makes us wonder: Why have we kneaded the problem when the solution was apparent?

When all is said and done, we have presented but one idea: that women who are treated hospitably, whose needs are considered, whose bodies are respected, whose mothering responsibilities are honored, will give birth more easily; that those who are challenged, restrained, distrusted, and treated indifferently will have more trouble with birth. We have only said that drugs and technology in birth, as in life, have proved to be poor substitutes for true, human attention.

It is peculiar to have to make a case for decency, to prove that prevailing birth practices are poor because they are disrespectful of nature and the needs of women who are becoming mothers, but it has been necessary: In recent years, the problem in birth has not been an absence of the solution, but in our inability to see the problem.

In birth, women have denied assault and absorbed pain. Clearly they have done so for the best of reasons—in the name of their children and for their own survival. The very urgency of responsibility may have stunned critical capacity. It is relatively easy, after all, to challenge prevailing practices when one risks only oneself; it is a far, far more serious undertaking to make challenges when one may be risking the welfare of one's child. We may be naturally conservative at birth.

It is unfortunate, then, that we must question accepted truths to consider the possibility that the safest, healthiest births are not those that are medically managed. We must relinquish unnecessary dependence on technology and reevaluate female reproductive capacity. We might even have to reassert the importance of parenting work. We must, in other words, take on the prevailing culture. It isn't easy, not only because it feels like it requires courage, but because it does, in fact, require looking at our own culture as a stranger might see it.

To switch from the medicalized image of birth to the natural one requires, in other words, a paradigm shift, an exchange of fields of perception. It is the difference between viewing human nature from a seat on a subway train one day and from a family farm the next. Because everything is changed, the contrast is literally unbelievable. Nevertheless, when the shift in field occurs, as it has in some institutions in America, the results are dramatic.

Pennsylvania Hospital made the transition. It began on a superficial level years ago. The administration heard women demanding that birth be made more normal and more family-centered and so appropriated a staff locker room, slipcovered it, and called it a birthing room.

The room, which is still in operation today, has the requisite birthing bed, a flowery bedspread, curtains at the window, a rocking chair, and wood furniture. On the other hand, it retained a number of medical appurtenances—oxygen and suction outlets in the wall (a state requirement), a plastic isolette for the baby, a metal scale, a warming light, a stand for IVs, a high, chrome-legged chair for the doctor. The space, like so many other birthing rooms in hospitals, is in competition with itself, as if undecided whether to be a delivery room or a motel room. One of the major interior-design flaws, Bruce Herdman commented, is that "they put a great big clock in front of the bed so that the patient could watch the clock and know exactly how often she was in tremendous pain." Stumped himself by the insensitivity, he said, "I don't know, labor rooms had to have clocks." High tech, apparently, is vaporous, and can seep under doors.

The next step—that of building a separate Birthing Suite run by midwives—sounds like a paradigm shift. The administration and some of the obstetricians realized that the institutional emphasis on high-tech care, exquisite as it had become, was a disservice to those women who did not require it. They began to investigate the possibility of offering a genuine low-tech service. To be sure, they operated in a climate amenable to change. Midwifery care was not a foreign concept in Philadelphia: Booth Maternity Center was there, the University of Pennsylvania had a graduate midwifery program, and Pennsylvania Hospital was the principal training site for the university's midwives. The principal obstetric practice at the hospital, headed by the department chairman, Ronald J. Bolognese, MD, employs two midwives. Valerie Jorgensen practices with a midwife.

For all of that, the commitment to build the Birthing Suite required a leap of imagination, and Herdman—who is engaging and humble—gives the credit for it to H. Robert Cathcart, who is president of the hospital. Cathcart is known for his humane leadership in hospital administration and his energetic support of nursing. He, Herdman, and some others went off to talk with Joyce Thompson, who heads the nurse-midwifery program at University of Pennsylvania; they met with Ruth Lubic, head of the Maternity Center Association in New York, and Kitty Ernst, president of National Association of Childbearing Centers; they learned about the excellent statistics reported by birth centers. "Once you've listened to those two [Lubic and Ernst], you don't have any choice about what you do," Herdman said. So it was that Pennsylvania Hospital decided to harvest the experience of midwives. They invited every Philadelphia midwife to a dinner to brainstorm the idea of a birthing suite in a high-tech hospital—where it should go, who would use it, etc. Herdman calls that consultation "essential" in their development of the program.

They located the Birthing Suite across the street from the major hospital complex, connected to it by an underground walkway—far enough, Herdman says, so that high tech can't seep under its doors. Richard Jennings, one of the very few male midwives in America and director of the suite, wears a baggy, tweedy coat as he shuffles around the peach-walled corridors. Being as he's about as severe as oatmeal, one is surprised to hear him describe his suspicions of the Pennsylvania Hospital plan for a midwife-run unit. He attended the meetings the hospital held for the city's midwives and listened to their concern about whether it could happen "the right way." When the hospital asked him to be the suite's director, he agreed only because he knew he could walk out and go back to independent practice (which included home birth) if the place turned out to be a sham—which is what everyone else expected.

"I was never tempted [to leave]," he said. "I really get treated well. . . . Everyone, from the administration on down, has been great to me."

After a year in operation, he reports, he's found that the Birthing Suite has not been troubled by medical intrusionaries. True, there have been the necessary misunderstandings and negotiations, but these have been manageable and Jennings, the other midwives, and the nursing staff have been free to provide the quality of personal care and family consideration that marks midwifery.

In the Birthing Suite, the environment is "naturally pleasant." The midwives are "technically skilled," but they are also "warm and interested in families." Women give birth—which Jennings describes as "passionate and basic"—without anesthetics, their babies rarely need resuscitation, the family can curl up in bed afterward with their babies. Nurses have found that it's quite possible to do tests—taking a blood sample from a newborn, for example—without ever removing the child from its parent's arms.

After a year in operation, the majority of nurses from Pennsylvania Hospital were choosing to have their babies in the Birthing Suite. The peri- and neonatologists were enthusiastic. Several of the specialist, high-risk obstetricians work to reduce risk factors in their patients and, whenever possible, refer them to the midwives for delivery. As for Jennings, he doesn't show a trace of cynicism. Sitting in an armchair in the lounge, looking across the street at the facade encasing that tubed and wired delivery room as if it were a foreign country, he says, half-apologizing for the emotion that creeps into his voice, "I feel I am involved in one of the few mysteries left in life . . . the power . . . the mystifying process . . ."

It might be said that it was the opening of the Birthing Suite at Pennsylvania Hospital that legitimized the hospital's claim to being state-of-the-art. The hospital continues to offer some of the most sophisticated high-risk care available in this country, but, opening the Birthing Suite implies an appreciation of the human and caring aspects of medicine and health as well as a mature rejection of the Faustian temptations of technology.

Pennsylvania Hospital, it seems, is beginning to master one of the major challenges of medical science in the later twentieth century: that is, to come to terms with the human capacity to save lives by miraculous intervention and, at the same time, to create a climate that reduces the need for them. In a sense, they go beyond *"primum non nocere"* or "first, do no harm." The birthing suite across the street from the high-tech hospital suggests that we are wise to invest in health creation. As if to say: First, do good.

Mothering Today's Mother

Edie Wonnel is founder and director of the Birth Center of Delaware in Wilmington. She's an excellent practitioner, having been initiated into midwifery the hard way—that is, by delivering babies in Harlem tenement homes some thirty years ago. She is also a mother; not only does she have four grown children, but she looks like she's basted a lot of turkeys. Wonnel provokes a sort of silly thought: that if we had taken those doctors who entered women's bedchambers so long ago and dropped them into a pot to simmer with the women who negotiated with them, we'd end up today with some perfectly aged mom 'n' doc practitioner like her. But then, we think, it's not such a ridiculous idea after all because the Birth Center does combine the best of two traditions. Wonnel requires clinical excellence in herself and her partner midwives: "The technical background . . . I want to see credentials. Where she studied. What she did . . . common sense . . . judgment." In the same people, she wants sensitivity: "The soft fuzzies. You have to be sensitive, accepting, trusting, warm, easy to be with, and confident in yourself as a person able to help somebody else."

In planning the Birth Center, Wonnel's purpose was to offer an appropriate, modern, hospitable setting for pregnant couples and families. About eight years ago, she bought a house one block from a hospital. When her proposal went for public hearings, she had the predictable challenges from the status quo: "Open this place and the gutters will be running with blood. Babies will die," a doctor proclaimed at one meeting. "Well, I don't see what the big deal is," countered a Veterans Administration physician, putting the thing into perspective, "We can airlift wounded soldiers off the battlefield. Why can't we transport a woman a block to the hospital?"

She wallpapered the parlor, put in a Murphy bed (for inevitable overbookings), installed some couches, lamps, plants, etc., and called it a waiting room. She redid the kitchen downstairs, put in another upstairs, added a living room, a fireplace, installed bathtubs, showers, and Jacuzzis, brought in her modest equipment—which is kept in ordinary chests-of-drawers—hung up her diplomas, found a partner, and opened. Six years later, she reports that 84 percent of the women who start at the Birth Center give birth without anesthetics, that only 3.7 percent of all her clients end up with cesareans; that only 11 percent have episiotomies and that mothers and babies don't die from birth.

But that's surface information, really, the outward signs of success. What makes the Birth Center of Delaware and others like it dynamic is the practical, human, and domestic sensibility informing them. Wonnel and the other midwives know their clients. The women are not from some tribe coming down out of the hills bearing tablets of original truths, but the very women we have been describing: women whose mothers were put out during birth, women who tend to feel safer with technology around them, women who were raised to venerate doctors, women who have to go back to work in a few weeks. As often as not, Wonnel says, leafing through her files, couples come to the center not because of some high commitment to natural birth but because they hate hospitals.

She works with them, starting with their basic perceptions. "The lack of confidence in their bodies," Wonnel says. "All the technology has . . . become ingrained in them as part of normal childbearing and, 'How can you have a baby without a fetal monitor? Doesn't everybody get a fetal monitor? Doesn't everybody get an IV?' . . . I think that's the big, gutsy issue. We have so convinced women that their bodies cannot do this without help." Thus each client, each couple must, in a sense, undergo that paradigm shift—release their inherited suspicions of women's reproductive capacity and somehow begin to believe in themselves and in the wisdom of nature. They must give up their culturally acquired dependence on technology. They must learn to think differently about themselves.

Assembled in the parlor waiting room, pregnant couples are taught that birth is very rarely an emergency. One of Wonnel's colleagues, Cynthia Oberdeck, uses a pathologic parallel to explain, "You don't just get pneumonia, you start with a cold and the cold gets worse and you get sicker and sicker. . . . It's the same with obstetrics. You don't just bleed or the baby doesn't just get bad, there are lots of things that push you in that direction and you begin to get symptoms." To help prevent emergencies, a pregnant woman or couple have a responsibility to be conscious of the quality of their pregnancy, to pay attention to what's going on inside them, and to ask questions.

The prevailing concept at the center is that one assists a woman best not by separating her from her body, but by giving her every opportunity to become better acquainted with it. "We are teaching self-help, self-confidence. We give the usual things on diet and exercise and changes in pregnancy and I do one class on monitoring pregnancy. I teach them how to take blood pressure, they do their own urine—what turning up a one-plus protein may mean, or sugar in your urine. . . . So, for example, if we have a mother at the end who has to be at home on bed rest, we can send her home with her own urine sticks . . . or blood pressure cuffs so her husband can take her blood pressure." During exams, they can feel where the baby's head or bottom is. They can listen to the baby's heartbeat with the stethoscope. Sensitivities enhanced, a couple can begin to trust their evaluation of their baby's liveliness.

Being gently touched, a couple learns in their bones and muscles what ordinary measures give comfort and settle pain—knowledge that will serve them well in the middle of the night when they are alone with a crying child. Feeling themselves cared for, they are better prepared to be able to soothe a child. Sensing the well-being that comes from being understood, they begin to learn one of the most important skills in nurturing a child.

The Birth Center prepares couples psychologically. They write up a birth plan not with the idea that birth will follow its prescription but, in part, so that they can anticipate their reactions to labor and birth. "One of the things in the birth plan," Cynthia says, "is how do you handle stress? How do you cope? . . . With first-time mothers, we kind of have them hypothesize about 'How will I be under stress?' . . . Some say, 'I get hysterical,' and we say, 'Whatever.' " Partners are invited to imagine how birth will be for them. At an orientation Cynthia showed slides. The father in the featured birth had taken his shirt off and was holding the new baby against his bare chest. "One of the prospective fathers said, 'I don't think I want to participate quite to that level.' . . . He was saying, people may get real organic, but that's not my thing. . . . He was saying, 'Do I have to be real funky?' I say, 'No.' " Edie says, "We love you no matter what you do."

In other words, they have the attitudes of home and family. In classes held at the center clients get acquainted with the place, its smells, rhythms, light switches, hallways, kitchen appliances, and bedrooms. They learn to know all the midwives. More important, perhaps, considering how short a time one is pregnant and laboring and how long one is a parent, is the opportunity to become acquainted with other couples. Friendships formed during the prenatal phase of pregnancy often deepen during the postpartum period when women and couples return to share their birth stories, to talk about the feelings of having a new baby, and to figure out the multitude of new problems they are facing. By this arrangement, couples who otherwise might be lonely for companionship during their new enterprise make natural connections.

More and more, Wonnel is deescalating the professional presence in birth and baby care. The midwives are there to educate, to watch for signs of complications, to manage them, and to be a guardrail during birth. They are not there to siphon off parental confidence, responsibility, or involvement. To the contrary, they invest in those qualities. People learn that they can take care of themselves and their babies without having years of medical education behind them.

Wonnel talks about offering a kind of buddy system, whereby experienced birthers accompany first-timers through their births, reminding us of the old days when women went to one another's homes at birth. She's working it out so that the nurse who teaches the postpartum classes says less and asks couples to say more— which reminds us of the advantages of the old neighborhood coffee klatches and how much essential knowledge and plain old comfort was passed on at them. She has it in mind to invite experienced parents to the baby-care classes so that new ones can take from the rich anecdotal stew. Thus couples, because they work forty- and fifty-hour weeks, because they are separated from extended families, because their activities are often child-free, because they live in neighborhoods where children are invisible, will suffer less from educational deprivation. They are enfolded, like Manuel's Suzie was, by those who know.

For grandparents she offers separate classes, taught by a grandmother/nurse so that the Twilight Sleep generation, the ones who are suspicious of birth, who followed bottle-feeding schedules and regimented toilet training, can learn where birth and baby care have come since they had their own children. Grandparents can ask questions without looking stupid or contrary in front of their children and sometimes they are invited to births. They often witness the primary reproductive act for the first time. They see what they weren't allowed to feel; they cry; they are proud; they are moved. They reclaim what was withheld from them. Birth stories are reborn—the great guiding power of myth is restored.

At the Birth Center of Delaware, in particular, the legacies of birth, of mothering, parenting, and family are being reconstructed. Drawing on the core traditions of women who were homemakers, defining the nourishing dynamics within them, Edie has translated them into an appropriate contemporary form. She has designed an institution that permits giving and taking, that invites one generation to share with another and makes caretaking more of a human and less of a speciality concern. Talking to one of her postpartum mothers, a New York City construction manager, one knows that Edie is not attempting to re-create an old, sentimentalized family form—the one in which Mom stayed at home with the kids and Dad went out to work. She doesn't seem to have any rules about who should be included in and/or excluded from intimacy or domesticity; she doesn't expect people to organize their personal lives or loyalties according to a designated structure. Neither does she require a woman, her partner, or her parents to be superhuman at birth. Quite the reverse, she understands that those who are taking up the responsibilities of family will prosper best if they are welcomed and given to. She emphasizes that at home one must be loved not on the basis of performance, but for one's being.

It might be that these birth-center births are far more important than their woundless statistics suggest. Wonnel and others like her, by behavior and attitude, are passing on ways of making family.

Restoring the Legacy

Doug Walker, a TV cameraman, was out to Penny's house to film part of a story on the Amish. He shuttled his equipment efficiently and unobstrusively while the reporter asked crisp questions. He must have been paying attention, however, because as we were standing around waiting for the mist to clear enough so he could get some shots of the farmland through the alder trees, he edged up to Penny and told her that his wife had had a baby with a midwife. "It was in a birth center," he said. "Do you know about those?" Well, she did, she said, but she'd like to hear his experience and they agreed that Doug would come out on the following Saturday with the baby. His wife had to work.

You can tell when a person's experienced in caring for a baby. There's no fumbling for the strings holding a bonnet on, no awkwardness with car-seat straps, booties, or sleeper snaps. The work gets done, the caregiver even talks to the infant, but they can carry on a conversation with another adult at the same time. Doug had all the easy moves with four-month-old Colleen; the only thing he hadn't overcome was the thrill of her. "Look at her thumb," he said, pulling back the fluffy trim on the sleeve of her sweater, "it's exactly the same as mine." He settled her in the corner of his arm so we could admire her sleeping and proceeded to tell his birth story, as women do, in one fell swoop.

Doug had given up on the idea of children. He and his first wife had had a stillborn child and their marriage didn't survive the loss. At thirty-seven, about the time he'd decided he would always be single, he met Kate, a teacher in an alternative school, and they married. "One of Kate's friends became very ill. She had a little one-year-old girl and no one to take care of her. So we took the baby in for a few months, I spent a lot of time looking out after her and she sort of adopted me and that was it. I was pie-eyed about her. After she went back to her mother, I couldn't get it out of my mind that I wanted a baby." Kate, whose fifteen-year-old daughter was living with her dad, wasn't so sure at first—having thought all that was behind her—but "I guess she couldn't help herself when she saw how crazy I was about that kid. Kate's a soft touch.

"I was a pest, all the way through the pregnancy. We went for an amniocentesis and the doctor finally had to push me aside so he could get in there and do his work. Then, what do I do? I see the needle and I get woozy. I have to leave the room. I'm thinking, if I get faint at the amnio, what good am I going to be at the birth?

"Of course, by that time, we'd already signed up with Mimi, the midwife. That was Kate's doing. I was torn, myself. My idea was that you get the best doctor in town, you have EKGs, EEGs, all those tests—probably because of the stillbirth. You know, Kate's not a communist or anything but she said that if she was going to have another baby, she was going to do it her way. Her first husband was sort of a jerk when he was younger, and so she'd been all alone when she had Samantha, her daughter, and they'd pushed her around quite a bit in the hospital. Anyway, since it was my idea to have the baby in the first place, I thought that the least I could do was to go to the birth center.

"Kate was into it. She takes me, her daughter, *and* her mother to the orientation. Samantha, naturally, wants to know why her mother can't have babies the way other women have them—like when they're much younger and in the hospital. She wasn't quite as contrary when the meeting was over, but all that's a long story. Anyway, she didn't come to the birth.

"As we walked in, Kate's mother was making sarcastic remarks about 'carrying this earth-mother thing a little too far. When I told my friends about what you were planning, they said they didn't know there were still hippies.' I suppose she was as terrified as I was. I guess she'd had a lot of trouble having babies. At one point, she took me aside and said, 'You'll make sure she sees a *real* doctor, won't you Doug?' Kate's mother is really OK and besides, this time I agreed with her. So, I nodded.

"When I met the midwives, they looked pretty straight and so I felt a little better. When I saw the oxygen tank in the cupboard I felt a little better yet. When I looked out the window above the cupboard where the oxygen tank is kept and saw the silhouette of the hospital, I felt much better. They tell us they have 'grandparents only' classes. Kate's mom says she'll go. 'Maybe I'll meet an attractive grandfather.' Like I said, she's OK.

"Still, I was twitchy as hell. And then, the way it happened wasn't what I expected. We thought there'd be this long, slow labor with plenty of time for sitting around the house, watching candles burn down, holding hands, playing music, seeing a couple of movies on the VCR. We kind of had it planned out. Instead, Kate wakes up at one-thirty in the morning, stumbles into the bathroom, comes out, says she "shot the plug [the mucus plug]," and crawls back into bed. "Go to sleep." Of course, that was a stupid thing to say. I know I'm supposed to be calm but I was dressed in three minutes and ready to launch. Good thing, too, I enjoy reminding her now, because within an hour she sounds like a bear.

"I call Mimi, who says something about a bath. I don't want to hear this, so I say, "Listen to this," and I put the receiver over to Kate's mouth just as she's letting go with this gale-force contraction. The midwife says we can come in if we want to.

"You know what really got to me. We drive up to the birth center and the porch light is on. There we are in the middle of the night, half dressed, carrying bundles, looking like a couple of immigrants, and when we get to the house, the porch light is on.

"We get Kate settled into the bedroom. Mimi checks her, says everything's fine, she's at three centimeters, and asks me if I want to listen to the baby's heartbeat. I can tell it's alive, which is a big relief, so I remember I'm supposed to call Kate's mom. I ask if there's time. Mimi says she thinks that would be fine. As I leave the room, she's rubbing Kate's back.

"The house was really quiet. And after I make the phone call, there's nothing for me to do, so I go sit by the bed and the midwife shows me how to do the massage. Making these long sweeping motions, I relax some myself. I take it upon myself to tell Kate to relax.

"She says—she wasn't very nice about it either, 'Doug, if you don't mind, I'm having a baby. Don't tell me what to do. I tell you: Just keep rubbing—harder. No, not there; lower down.'

"After that, I behave myself. I forget about my anxiety. I'm watching Kate and I'm so impressed. I can't imagine doing what she's doing. I help her into the bathroom, where Mimi's got a warm Jacuzzi bath going. She leaves us alone and I sit on the side of the tub and dribble warm water over Kate's shoulders. I can't do enough for her.

"Kate's mom arrives about then, and the contractions start getting stronger. Seems to me they're making the waves, not the Jacuzzi. Her mom stands by the tub through one of those. When it's passed, Kate reaches for her mom's hand, holds it to her face, and says, 'Hi, Mom.' There's tears in her mom's eyes, so she gets a little brusque and says, 'I'll be doing my cross-stitching in the living room if you need me.'

"One more contraction and Kate announces that she wants out

of the tub—now. I get Mimi, who wraps her in a towel to walk her back to the bedroom. As she's walking down the hallway, she looks back over her shoulder and waves at her mom. 'Go talk to her for a minute, Doug,' she commands.

"By this time, I'm acting like a love slave, so I dutifully go in and sit down in this big leatherette lounger they have there. I think it must be for the men who have already had five or six children, because it feels way too big for me. Anyway, I tell Kate's mom that Mimi said it would only be another hour or so and that Kate wanted me to ask how she was doing.

" 'Well,' she said, 'I was just thinking about that. You know when Kate had Samantha, I told them not to call me until after she was born—that's an indication of how much I like the idea of worrying through one my daughter's labors. So, in the first place, I'm pretty impressed with myself for being here at all.'

"So I told her I was real glad she showed up and I knew that Kate was too. She nodded curtly, the way my mother does when she's telling me, 'You should be.'

" 'I'm glad you appreciate it,' she went on, 'because now that I am here, I have to say I hate to see my children suffer. I hated it when they were young and stepped on a damned bee or something; I can't say I like it much better now.

" 'When I was standing there by the bathtub, I was thinking about how I used to stand by the tub when Kate was a baby—the steam, the dew on her forehead. You know, there's a strand of her hair that has curled down when her hair got wet just the same way ever since she was two.'

" 'Is that right?' I said, feeling pretty stupid.

" 'Well, you probably don't want to hear all this, but when I was standing by the tub and I saw that look come over her face—when she had the contractions, you know—I almost reached over and tried to pick her up, wet and all, as I would have done thirty-six years ago, so I could comfort her, hold her in my arms, as if I could suck the pain out of her and into me.'

" 'That's kind of how I was feeling,' I said.

" 'But, you know, I couldn't have done that,' she continued. 'I don't mean in the physical sense, but something else. I can't describe it. Seeing her there, watching her face working through the contraction, it would have been wrong for me to pick her up. I would have been messing things up. She was so beautiful, so complete, so self-possessed, so strong. I don't know the words.'

"She looked down at her handwork. I did too.

" 'I am awe-struck, Doug,' she said, looking me straight in the eye. 'Proud. Proud of myself for having my daughter grow up and be the way she is, in there, right now. Maybe I feel complete. Maybe I understand something I didn't before. I feel kind of deferential.'

"We were both too choked up to talk after that. So we sat there for a couple of minutes and stared at the floor. Fortunately, Mimi came out and said that Kate wanted to know where I was, so I went back in to Kate. 'Your mother's awfully proud of you,' I said. 'She was getting pretty sappy about it.' Kate, who was going under again, smiled.

"Toward the end, Kate had her arms around my neck. I was soothing her, stroking her, and holding her. I felt so close. I even whispered to her that I wanted to make love to her—It wasn't that I would have or meant to—it's just that I felt that bound up with her.

"Colleen was born while Kate was hanging from my neck. She dug her fingernails into my flesh. I looked down and saw Mimi's hands appearing and then, it seemed like all at once, the baby was in them. I had tears streaming down my face. I was laughing and crying at the same time. Colleen had all this squirmy hair and she let out the tiniest cry. Mimi handed her to me with all the goop on her and I never even thought about it. She was so pink. She opened her eyes for the first time in her life right there in my arms. I thought she was the most beautiful thing I had ever seen. There was something about that, holding her just the way she was.

"After a bit, Mimi took the baby and put it to Kate's breast. She nursed a little and Kate pushed out the placenta. I wiped the blood off Kate's legs. I didn't even think about, about what I was touching or doing. It was absolutely natural—I just wanted Kate to be comfortable.

"Mimi had the bed cleaned up, a fresh gown on Kate, the baby checked, washed, and dressed before we knew it. And the three of us were curled up together there on the bed when Kate's mom came in. She didn't say anything. She didn't need to. We stayed there for the longest time, not saying anything, just watching Colleen breathe. I never felt anything like that in my life."[1]

There are 132 freestanding birth centers in America today. In them, birth is safer and healthier than in any other setting. In them a woman and those who are with her can experience that eruption of power that accompanies the arrival of a new life. In them a family can nourish the bonds that will sustain them. In them ordinary humans may feel the pulse of the everlasting source of life.

We would do well to imitate them whenever we can. It seems like the least we can do for the people who will be caring for our young.

Epilogue

THERE WERE many times when we were writing this book when the facts tempted us to say that sexism was, in fact, the underlying cause of all the destruction at birth. A sexism so profound that it would not be satisfied until women were reproductively neutered and until their traditional mothering work—because it was woman's work—was thoroughly discredited. One single event prevented us from taking up the interpretation.

We were in the process of outlining the book in the fall of 1987. Penny's husband, Rich, had been out poking around in local land affairs, as he liked to do, and he came home with the news that the state of Pennsylvania was planning to build a four-lane road through the very heart of the Amish country. Since this valley is blanketed with some of the most exceptional farming soil in the world, since the amount of rain makes irrigation unnecessary, and since the people who farm it are considered to be among the world's finest farmers, we were nonplussed.

Standing on Penny and Rich's porch, overlooking the abundance below, we reacted as might be supposed. We made sarcastic remarks about the stupidity of planners who wanted to bury farmland that was as close as this was to so many city people who needed to eat. We then seized on the irony of taking land from the pacifist Amish so that transport to and from the growing defense industry around Lancaster could be eased. Seeing the brusque, burnished color of drying corn stalks, we were soon shuddering at the thought of destroying the beauty of the place. We could feel, as surely as if we were alfalfa leaves and marigold petals, a film of automobile and truck exhaust suffocating our skin. It took us several days to grow into our passion.

As we grew accustomed to it, however, working on the outline of the book as we did, it occurred to us that there might well be a parallel between the thoughtless proposal to scar this fertile land and the similarly thoughtless scarring of women at reproductive work. As we contemplated the road proposal by the state of Pennsylvania to pave the valley, it seemed to us that obstetricians were behaving no differently from society at large. Just as the state was unfamiliar with the subtle interdependencies between good farmers and their land, so medical culture neglected the natural and human dynamics of birth. We realized that in America we have not only assaulted reproduction in women, but that we have done the same to men. We have, until recently, routinely cut the sensitive foreskin on baby boys' penises without anesthesia. It is as if we are terrified of our reproductive capacities—or our ignorance thereof—and must mutilate them in order to tame them.

It seemed plausible to us, therefore, that the destruction of women at birth may have less to do with the fact that they are women than with the fact that birth is a natural and generative act. And nature, with her dark side, has frightened us, made us want to control her, manipulate and command her.

The story that Doug came out to film was about the citizens' challenge to the building of the road through the heart of Amish farmland. Since then, the governor of Pennsylvania decreed that it would never be, and that is good. His decision made us think of the American College of Obstetricians and Gynecologists when they said, essentially: Don't do cesareans just because you've done them before, which was also good.

On the other hand, as time went by, it became clear that the proposal of a road through Amishland was merely the symptom of a much larger underlying problem. The farmland here is still in jeopardy from housing developers, mall builders, and industrial planners. Similarly, the College's urging avoidance of unnecessary cesareans does not correct for the underlying dynamics leading to cesareans and other forms of wounding births.

Our behavior at birth, therefore, seems to us to be but one manifestation of our imperfect understanding about the nature of the earth and the nature of nature. On the one hand, that can cause us to despair: Perhaps we will not stop wounding women until we have given up debilitating the earth. On the other, we can be hopeful: As we become more sophisticated in understanding how to tend this planet, which gives us life, it will be natural for us to tend women well when they give birth.

References

INTRODUCTION

1. Penny Armstrong and Sheryl Feldman, *A Midwife's Story* (New York: Arbor House, 1986). Also in paperback (New York: Fawcett Books, 1988).
2. See note 1, Part One: The Nature of Birth, page 265.
3. Adrienne Rich, *Of Woman Born,* Tenth Anniversary Edition (New York: W. W. Norton, 1986), p. 139.
4. Ibid., p. 169.

ON THE POWER

1. With one exception, which we note, we have not used the real names of the men and women whose birth stories we tell.
2. The fetal monitor is a machine used for tracking the baby's heartbeat during labor. It has two sensor devices that are placed on the mother's belly and held there by a strap around her body. Wires connect the sensors to

a machine that records the baby's heartbeat in relation to contractions. The information is printed out on graph paper.

PART ONE: THE NATURE OF BIRTH

INTRODUCTION

1. *National statistics:*
The National Center of Health Statistics does not record drug use in birth. Although the epidural is just one of the drugs used, we used it as an indicator of general trends. The number we use for reference, 60 percent, is likely to be conservative; furthermore, it varies tremendously. In some hospitals, it is as high as 90 percent, in others it is not used at all. This range indicates that it is the place of birth, not the woman at birth, that most determines whether an epidural is "needed." At a presentation for the International Childbirth Education Association in August 1988, Margery Simchak, BSN, RN, argued that there is a correlation between the arrival of anesthesiologists in a hospital and an escalation in the epidural rate.

We note that there is a correlation between use of the epidural and forceps deliveries. Determinative studies have not been made, but one observer estimates that the risk of forceps delivery is increased by five times when a woman has an epidural. (Michel Odent, *Birth Reborn* [New York: Pantheon Books, Random House, 1984], p. xvii).

In 1988, episiotomies were reported in 61 percent of all hospital-based vaginal births. "However, it might be worth noting how these data were obtained. The short stay records from 418 hospitals were surveyed throughout the US, using discharge summary and face sheets. . . . however labor and delivery records are not screened to check for disparity. Because an episiotomy is usually considered a routine procedure, there may be physicians who do not document it on the summary sheets. Lay literature and speakers in the field of childbirth have suggested that over 80 percent of the childbearing women in the US have an episiotomy." (Jean Campen, "Statistics Corner," *International Journal of Childbirth Education* [May 1988], 13.)

The National Center of Health Statistics reported a 24.1 percent cesarean section rate in 1986. From the same source, the U.S. perinatal mortality rate in 1986 was 10.4 per thousand—a number that is influenced by the poor distribution of prenatal care in this country.

Penny's statistics:
My statistics are based on ten years of experience. They include everyone accepted for care. My intrapartum transfer rate—that is, after labor has begun—was 1 percent. The perinatal mortality rate, when corrected for

gross congenital anomalies incompatible with life, e.g., anacephaly, was zero. The total number of births, 1,246.

I collected my statistics for the Pennsylvania Chapter of the American College of Nurse Midwives Peer Review Committee for 1987–88. Of the 129 pregnancies I attended during that year, 119 were delivered at home, 10 were transferred before the onset of labor, and 5 of those transferred had cesarean sections. There were 3 perinatal deaths in the transfer group, all attributable to gross congenital anomalies. In the 119 births that began at home there were no transfers and the perinatal mortality in this group was zero. There were no third- or fourth-degree lacerations in the home-birth group, and the episiotomy rate was zero.

2. A certified nurse-midwife is an individual educated in the two disciplines of nursing and midwifery, who possesses evidence of certification according to the requirements of the American College of Nurse-Midwifery. Nurse-midwifery practice is the independent management of care of essentially normal newborns and women—antepartum, intrapartum, postpartum, and/or gynecologically, occurring within a health-care system which provides for medical consultation, collaborative management or referral.

State requirements for nurse-midwifery must also be met. Currently there are 3300 certified nurse-midwives in America. They serve 4 percent of American woman at birth.

THE NATURE OF POWER

1. Armstrong and Feldman, *Midwife's Story*.
2. Grace Kaiser tells about her experiences among the Amish in *Dr. Frau: A Woman Doctor Among the Amish* (Intercourse, Pennsylvania: Good Books, 1986).
3. As a precautionary measure, hospital protocols often disallow women from taking food or drink during labor; instead they will give her glucose intravenously. The reasoning behind the protocol is that a woman might have to be put out instantly, that is, by having her inhale an anesthetic gas. A hazard of this intervention is Mendelson's Syndrome, which occurs when gastric contents are vomited and subsequently inhaled secondary to the relaxation which occurs with anesthesia. Although the sequence of events is rare, the results can be deadly.

The National Center for Health Statistics does not keep numbers on Mendelson's Syndrome. Ruben et al reported a maternal death rate in Georgia of 59.3 deaths per 100,000 cesarean section deliveries during 1975–1976. In three of the 9 cesarean-attributed deaths, the women had clinical courses consistent with Mendelson's. This is compared with 18.8 deaths per 100,000 live births for all methods of delivery in Georgia. (G. L. Rubin, H. Peterson, R. Rochat, et al., "Maternal Death After Cesarean Section in Georgia." *Am J Obstet Gynecol,* 1981, 139, pp. 681–685.)

I made a different analysis of the risks. In the first place, there is one study that suggests that IV glucose may decrease the threshold of pain perception and the maximum level of pain tolerated. (G. K. Marley, A. D. Morradian, A. S. Levine, J. E. Morley, "Mechanisms of Pain in Diabetic Peripheral Neuropathy." *Am J Med,* 1984; 77: pp. 79–82.) Furthermore, the IV limits a woman's movements and, in that, restricts her labor. It also communicates to her that she is a patient—an ill person rather than a healthy, birthing one. Both these factors increase the likelihood of cesarean. Since it is rare that indications for a section cannot be picked up in time for a woman to have an epidural, which is effective in five to fifteen minutes, since there are hazards of cesarean section (see note 11 under "Discouraging Birth," below), I believe that the less risky protocol is one that allows a laboring woman some nourishment.

4. The term *fetus ejection reflex* was first proposed in 1966 by Niles Newton, Donald Foshee, and Michael Newton. "Experimental Inhibition of Labor Through Environmental Disturbance," *Obstet Gynecol,* 1966, 27, pp. 371–77.

5. Odent, *Birth Reborn,* 13.

6. The hormonal wisdom does continue after birth, which we will not attempt to explain here, but there are studies that indicate that their free flow after birth—at that point, estrogen and prolactin—stimulate maternal behavior such as grooming and cuddling, which the mother and no doubt the child experience with pleasure. (Odent, *Birth Reborn,* p. 15.)

7. If the animal mother is frightened late in the birth process, the body reacts by hastening birth. Having expelled the newborn, the mother may be able to protect it by fight or flight. In one speech, Odent recalled how home birth practitioners used to call for forceps when they saw a woman's energy flagging near the end of birth. Her fear of them was thought to provoke the necessary surge.

THE INNER NATURE OF BIRTH

1. He also reduced the perinatal mortality rate at Pithiviers. Under Odent's leadership, it dropped from 29 infant deaths per thousand to 10 per thousand. (Odent, *Entering the World: The Demedicalization of Childbirth* [New York: New American Library, 1984], p. 116.)

2. Odent, *Birth Reborn,* p. 118.

DISCOURAGING BIRTH

1. These statistics are found in an unpublished document put out by the National Association of Childbearing Centers (NACC). Entitled "Information Concerning the Quality of Nurse-Midwifery Care," it is available from NACC, RD1, Box 1, Perkionmenville, PA 18074.

2. From an interview with Dr. Eisenstein and from a report in *The Clarion*, 1989, vol. 6, no. 4, p. 13. *The Clarion* is the newsletter for the Cesarean Prevention Movement. See note 6 below.

3. Noted from Stevenson's report at the First International Home Birth Conference, London, 1987.

4. Home Birth Service of Los Angeles. Numbers provided by Deborah Frank, CNM.

5. J. Rooks, N. Weatherby, E. Ernst, S. Stapleton, D. Rosen, A. Rosenfield, "Outcomes of Care in Birth Centers," *New England Journal of Medicine*, 1989, 321, pp. 1804–1811.

6. For information about CPM or to receive its newsletter, *The Clarion*, write P.O. Box 152, Syracuse, New York 13210 or call 315-424-1942.

7. Vaginal birth after cesarean section (VBAC) became possible with the advent of the transverse lower uterine segment incision, which, should it rupture, does not carry with it the high maternal and infant mortality and morbidity associated with rupture of the older, classical or vertical incision. Before the change to transverse incisions, the standard of care was, "Once a cesarean, always a cesarean." (B. E. Finley, C. E. Gibbs, "Emergency Cesarean Delivery in Patients Undergoing a Trial of Labor with a Transverse Lower Segment Scar." *Am J Obstet Gynecol,* 1986, 155, pp. 936–39.)

8. See Stephen A. Meyers and Norbert Gleicher, "A Successful Program to Lower Cesarean-Section Rates." *New England Journal of Medicine,* 1988, 319, pp. 1511–16. To the credit of those who participated in the study, it was undertaken in defiance of financial advantage. "Neither physicians nor the institution had financial incentives to decrease the cesarean section rates. In fact the opposite was the case. The hospital's reimbursement for vaginal deliveries is approximately $3,000 lower than for deliveries by cesarean-section. Also, physicians' fees are usually $250 to $500 lower for vaginal deliveries. Expenses for liability insurance changed little. Revenues for both the staff and the hospital . . . decreased as a result of the initiative" (p. 1516).

9. Janice Kaplan, "Do Cesareans Save Lives?" *Parents* (January 1988), p. 88.

10. Associated Press report carried in Seattle *Post-Intelligencer,* October 27, 1988, p. A-5. The American College of Obstetricians and Gynecologists is less directive. They recommend counseling a woman for VBAC. Excerpting from "Guidelines for Vaginal Delivery After Cesarean Birth," ACOG Committee Opinion (October 1988), No. 64: "The concept of routine repeat cesarean birth should be replaced by a specific indication for a subsequent abdominal delivery, and in the absence of a contraindication, a woman with one previous cesarean delivery with a low transverse incision should be counseled and encouraged to attempt labor in her current pregnancy." Similarly, "A woman with two or more previous cesarean deliveries with

low transverse incisions who wishes to attempt vaginal birth should not be discouraged from doing so in the absence of contraindications."

11. Nancy Wainer Cohen and L. J. Estner, *Silent Knife* (South Hadley, Massachusetts: Bergen and Garvey Publishers, 1983), p. 30, cite The National Institutes of Child Health and Human Development, Draft Report of the Task Force on Cesarean Childbirth (Bethesda, Md: NIH, Sept. 1980). From the same source: "A cesarean delivery is a major operative procedure and as such is associated with many complications leading to maternal morbidity that are never encountered in a vaginal delivery."

For an excellent, readable discussion of the hazards of cesarean from a medical point of view (and how to avoid one), see Mortimer Rosen and Lillian Thomas, *The Cesarean Myth* (New York: Penguin Books, 1989). Rosen, professor and chairman of the department of obstetrics and gynecology at Columbia University and director of obstetrics and gynecology in the Sloan Hospital for Women of the Presbyterian Hospital of New York City, says, "The fact is that the mother who undergoes a cesarean is at much higher risk of dying than the woman who gives birth vaginally; twice the risk for an elective cesarean; four times the risk for an emergency cesarean" (p. 9).

Statistics on the risks of cesarean section vary. The risk of maternal death is reported as being between two and twenty-six times higher for women having cesarean section than for those who deliver vaginally, depending on where the study was conducted. Two studies that report a twelve times higher risk are D. Lehmann, W. Mabie, J. Miller, M. Pernoll, "The Epidemiology and Pathology of Maternal Mortality: Charity Hospital of Louisiana in New Orleans," *Obstet Gynecol,* 1987, 69, pp. 833–44 and P. Moldin, K-H. Hokegard and T. F. Nielsen, "Cesarean Section and Maternal Mortality in Sweden, 1973–1979," *Acta Obstet Gynecol Cand,* 1984, 63, pp. 7-11. Another study reports that 50 percent of all new mothers delivered by cesarean section have some serious illness such as infection or hemorrhage. S. G. Doering, "Unnecessary Cesarean: Doctor's Choice and Patient's Dilemma," *Compulsory Hospitalization* (no. 48, ch. 2), 1, pp. 145–52.

Cohen and Estner argue that deaths attributable to cesarean section are "notoriously underreported" (p. 29).

12. Albert Haverkamp, MD, clinical professor of obstetrics and gynecology and preventive medicine at the University of Colorado Health Science Center, is quoted in *Parents* magazine (January 1988), p. 88. The article states, "He points out that Denver General Hospital has a very low cesarean rate—about 13 percent—and one of the lower rates of perinatal mortality in Colorado. 'Those facts aren't directly related,' he says, 'but it does show that after a certain point, doing a lot of cesareans doesn't mean you're saving babies.' "

13. These quotes come out of the same article in *Parents* (Ibid). More completely, it reads, "There's also new evidence that babies benefit from the actual process of labor. Researchers in Sweden have found that babies born after labor have higher levels of stress hormones in their blood than babies born by elective cesarean. These hormones—called catecholamines—help a baby's lungs mature, regulate body temperature, and send blood to the brain and heart. This may partially explain why cesarean babies are at a far great risk of suffering from symptoms of respiratory distress than babies who are born vaginally."

The 1985 edition of *Williams Obstetrics* (p. 868) observes: "Certainly, maternal and perinatal mortality and morbidity are typically higher with cesarean delivery, in part because of the complication that led to the cesarean section and in part because of the increased risks inherent in the abdominal route of delivery."

PART TWO: LEGACIES

REMEMBERING: THE GREAT EMERGENCY

1. Margaret Yourcenar, *Souvenirs Pieux,* Elaine Marks, trans. Epigraph in Judith Walzer Leavitt, *Brought to Bed: Childbearing in America, 1750–1950* (New York: Oxford University Press, 1986), p. 2. Leavitt gives us plenty of non-French examples of the fear women had about childbirth prior to the advent of modern medicine. She summarizes: "Women knew that if procreation did not kill them, it could maim them for life" (p. 28). We, apparently like Leavitt, found this Yourcenar quote particularly striking.
2. Margaret Mead and Niles Newton, "Cultural Patterning of Perinatal Behavior" in Stephen A. Richardson and Alan F. Guttmacher, eds., *Childbearing—Its Social and Psychological Aspects* (Baltimore: Williams and Wilkins Company, 1967), p. 192.
3. Leavitt, *Brought to Bed,* pp. 89–90. We've relied heavily in this chapter on *Brought to Bed.* The history is unique in that it draws on the journals and letters of women. Leavitt convincingly demonstrates that women had far more to do with decision-making in childbirth than they have generally been credited with.
4. Ibid., p. 93.
5. Ibid., p. 97.
6. Ibid., p. 101.
7. Ibid., p. 125.
8. Ibid., p. 51.
9. Ibid., p. 52.
10. Ibid., p. 25.

11. Paul Starr, *The Social Transformation of American Medicine* (New York: Basic Books, 1982).

12. Leavitt, *Brought to Bed,* p. 184.

13. Ibid. p. 179.

14. Ibid., pp. 186–87.

15. Ibid., p. 188.

16. Margot Edwards and Mary Waldorf, *Reclaiming Birth* (Trumansburg, New York: The Crossing Press, 1984), p. 13.

17. NACC "Information Concerning the Quality of Nurse-Midwifery Care" takes these figures from M. Laird, "Report on the Maternity Center Association Clinic, NY, 1931–1951," *Am J Obstet Gynecol,* 1961, 81, pp. 395–402.

18. Edwards, *Reclaiming Birth,* p. 9.

19. Ibid., p. 11.

20. NACC "Information Concerning the Quality of Nurse-Midwifery Care" cites T. Montgomery, "A Case for Nurse-Midwives," *Am J Obstet Gynecol,* 1969, 105, p. 3 and M. Meglen, "A Prototype of Health Services for Quality of Life in a Rural Community," *Bulletin of Nurse-Midwifery,* Nov. 1972, xvii, 4, pp. 103–113.

21. David N. Danforth, *Obstetrics and Gynecology,* 4th ed. (Philadelphia: Harper & Row, Publishers, 1982), p. 3.

22. For further reading on the history of midwifery, see Judy Litoff, *American Midwives, 1860 to Present* (Westport, Connecticut: Greenwood Press, 1978); chapters two and three in Barbara Ehrenreich and Deirdre English, *For Her Own Good* (Garden City, New York: Anchor Press/Doubleday, 1979); Richard W. Wertz and Dorothy C. Wertz, *Lying-In: A History of Childbirth in America* (New York: Schocken Books, 1979); the chapter "Hands of Flesh, Hands of Iron" in Adrienne Rich, *Of Woman Born* (New York: W. W. Norton, 1976, 1986); and Margot Edwards and Mary Waldorf, *Reclaiming Birth* (Trumansburg, New York: The Crossing Press, 1984).

HINDSIGHT

1. DeLee himself revised his opinions about delivery. His view of the preventive use of forceps "to protect the fetus from the crushing force of the pelvis" modified. In a 1938 interview, he said, when asked about the issue: "I wish I hadn't done it." Madeleine Shearer, editor of *Birth,* reviewing *Power and the Profession of Obstetrics* (Winter 1985), vol. 12, no. 4, p. 252.

REMEMBERING: WHAT MOTHER TOLD US

1. Betty Friedan, *The Feminine Mystique* (New York: Laurel Books/Dell, 1983), p. 121.

2. Leavitt, p. 128.
3. Ibid., p. 130.
4. Ibid., p. 136.
5. To distinguish this quote from the others immediately above, we note that it came from one of our interviews. The grandmother is describing a fifties birth.
6. From an interview with Charlotte Houde, CNM, describing her experience in a Portland, Maine hospital in the early sixties.
7. For this account, Sheryl thanks her friend Jacqueline Page. We should note that it is not Jackie, but Sheryl, who must take the responsibility for commenting that Mike Page (also a friend) has "lost all sense of proportion" from time to time.
8. Interview by authors, 1988.

REMEMBERING: THE INNER LEGACY

1. Jay S. Rosenblatt, "Social Environmental Factors Affecting Reproduction and Offspring in Infrahuman Mammals." Stephen A. Richardson, Ph.D., and Alan F. Guttmacher, eds., *Childbearing—Its Social and Psychological Aspects* (Williams and Wilkins, 1967), p. 164.
2. In this section, all quotes but this one are from Kitzinger's letter (January 6, 1988). This comes from her "Some Women's Experience of Epidurals: A Descriptive Study (London: The National Childbirth Trust and Sheila Kitzinger, 1987), p. 23.
3. While acknowledging that British midwifery education did not emphasize psychological factors and comfort/support measures, many British midwives told me that the hospital I trained at was particularly impoverished in this regard. They encouraged me to seek out members of the fledgling Association of Radical Midwives (ARM) who were working for more continuity and greater flexibility in care. Today ARM and the Association of Independent Midwives continue to support those goals.

PART THREE: PERPETUATING THE LOSS

THE OBSTETRICIAN'S CULTURE

1. *American Baby* (May 1988), p. 131.
2. The Report of the National Commission to Prevent Infant Mortality, "Death Before Life: The Tragedy of Infant Mortality" (Switzer Builder, Room 2006, 330 C Street, S. W., Washington D.C. 20201, August 1988), p. 11.
3. All quotes from *Williams Obstetrics* are from Jack A. Pritchard, Paul

C. MacDonald, Norman F. Gant, 17th ed. (Norwalk, Connecticut: Appleton-Century-Crofts, 1985).

4. Diony Young and Beth Shearer prepared the report on "Crisis in Obstetrics: The Management of Labor," a conference sponsored by the Department of Obstetrics and Gynecology of the College of Physicians and Surgeons of Columbia University and Presbyterian Hospital in New York, which appeared in the newsletter *The Midwife Advocate*, P.O. Box 237, Newtonville, MA 02160 (Fall & Winter 1987–88), vol. 4, nos. 3–4, pp. 2–3.

5. From one of our interviews.

6. Amy Roselle is not this resident's real name. Fearing reprisal, she preferred not to be identified.

7. Diana Scully, *Men Who Control Women's Health: The Miseducation of Obstetrician-Gynecologists* (Boston: Houghton Mifflin, 1980), pp. 104–5.

8. Ibid., p. 87.

9. Ibid., p. 105.

10. Ibid., p. 91.

11. Lynn Payer, *Medicine and Culture: Varieties of Treatment in the United States, England, West Germany, and France* (New York. Henry Holt and Company, 1988), p. 131.

12. Scully, *Men Who Control*, p. 118.

13. Ellen Ruppel Shell, "How to Talk to Your Doctor." *American Health* (February 1987), p. 84.

14. Steven Locke and Douglas Colligan, *The Healer Within* (New York: Mentor/New American Library, 1986), pp. 26–7.

15. Ibid., p. 19.

16. Ibid., p. 28.

17. Ronni Sandroff, "When the Obstetrician Says No," *Health* (November 1987), p. 54.

18. Payer, *Medicine and Culture*, p. 134.

THE MIDWIFE'S CULTURE

1. In 1982, the American College of Obstetricians and Gynecologists and the American College of Nurse-Midwives issued a joint statement supporting the concept of cooperative practice.

2. Quotes that follow are from Helen Varney, *Nurse-Midwifery*, ed. (Boston: Blackwell Scientific Publications, 1980 and 1987).

3. We chose to quote Paddy O'Brien's *Birth and Our Bodies* (London: Pandora, 1986), p. 40, primarily because it's so gently written. Unfortunately, the book is not available in the United States. Americans need not despair: They have Elizabeth Noble's excellent *Essential Exercises for the Childbearing Year* (Boston: Houghton Mifflin, 1976). Noble's *Childbirth with Insight* (Boston: Houghton Mifflin, 1983) is also an excellent resource. In it she explains the philosophy that informs her principles of childbirth.

4. Barbara K. Rothman clearly explains the risks of amniocentesis in *The Tentative Pregnancy* (New York: Penguin Books, 1987), p. 219.

Chorionic villi biopsy, which can be done as early as the seventh week in pregnancy, has been introduced as an answer to the concerns about amniocentesis. Enthusiasts cite the fact that the testing can be done as early as the seventh week in pregnancy. By comparison, one must wait until twenty weeks for the amniocentesis. Unfortunately, chorionic villi biopsy cannot entirely replace amniocentesis. It also has problems of its own. For a discussion, see *Tentative Pregnancy*, pp. 217–228.

5. For a discussion of risks attributable to ultrasound see R. Mole, "Possible Hazards of Imaging and Doppler Ultrasound in Obstetrics," *Birth-Special Supplement* (1986), pp. 23–33.

6. *Tentative Pregnancy*, pp. 104–5. The major concern of Rothman's book is the relationship between a woman's emotional state and technology. Filled with case studies and thoughtful analyses of them, *Tentative Pregnancy* is an excellent source for understanding the emotional ramifications of diagnostic procedures.

A VISIBILITY TALE

1. Wendy Savage, *A Savage Enquiry: Who Controls Childbirth?* (London: Virago Press, 1986), p. 168.

2. Elizabeth links her postpartum depression to the disrespect shown her by the hospital staff at labor and birth. Her opinion, however, cannot be verified by research on postpartum depression, mainly because it is inadequate. According to Carol Dix's *The New Mother Syndrome: Coping with Postpartum Stress and Depression,* American psychiatry does not classify postpartum depression as a mental illness. A woman's postpartum problems are attributed to latent conditions. Dix, who was a sufferer herself, suggests that the hormonal, neurohormonal, and biochemical changes during labor and birth may be significant factors in the condition. Others hypothesize that the woman who is brutalized and/or negated during a primary reproductive event has every reason to feel depressed.

Fortunately, awareness of the multifaceted problem of postpartum depression is slowly increasing and more and more practitioners and organizations are acknowledging the need for effective intervention in the form of both medical treatment (it is treatable) and emotional support. For resources, check with your local mental health center or contact: Depression After Delivery, P.O. Box 1282, Morrisville, PA 19607. Phone: 206-295-3994.

3. Savage, *Enquiry,* p. 119.

4. Ibid., p. 160.

5. Ibid., p. 93.

RECONCILIATIONS

1. Maureen Sayres, et al., "Pregnancy During Residency," *The New England Journal of Medicine* (February 13, 1986), 314, 7, p. 419.
2. Ibid., p. 421.
3. Ibid., p. 420.
4. Ibid., p. 421.
5. Ibid.
6. Ibid.
7. Alice Miller's *Thou Shalt Not Be Aware* (New York: Farrar Straus & Giroux, 1984) presents a convincing analysis of the transfer of emotional and behavioral patterns from one generation to the next. Following Miller, it seems reasonable to hypothesize that a similar, although shallower, transfer of attitudes might take place between caregiver and pregnant/laboring woman, given her vulnerable emotional state.
8. Perri Klass, "Anatomy and Destiny" *Ms* (July/August 1987), p. 66.
9. Ibid., p. 192.
10. Judith Rooks and J. Eugene Haas, "Nurse-Midwifery in America," A Report of the American College of Nurse-Midwives Foundation, 1522 K Street, N.W., Suite 1120, Washington, D.C. 20005.
11. Joyce Thompson, "Nurse-Midwifery Care: 1925–1984" in Harriet H. Wenley, Joyce T. Fitzpatrick, Roma Lee Taunton, eds., *Annual Review of Nursing Research* (1968) 4, p. 167.
12. Ibid., p. 169.
13. Ibid., p. 163.
14. Jacqueline Fawcett, "On Research and the Journal of Nurse-Midwifery: A Clinician's Viewpoint." *Journal of Nurse Midwifery* (March/April 1980), vol. 25, no. 3, p. 3.
15. Lisa L. Paine, R. G. Payton, and T. R. Johnson, "Ausculated FHR Accelerations: Part I: Accuracy and Documentation." *Journal of Nurse-Midwifery* (1986), vol. 31, no. 2, pp. 68–72. "Auscultated FHR Accelerations: Part II: An Alternative to the Nonstress Test, Ibid., pp. 73–77.
16. Some of Roberts's work can be found in Joyce Roberts et al., "The Descriptive Analysis of Involuntary Bearing-down Efforts During the Expulsive Phase of Labor," JOGNN (February 1987), pp. 48–55. Susan McKay and Joyce Roberts, "Second Stage Labor: What Is Normal?" JOGNN (April 1985), pp. 101–6. Joyce Roberts, "Alternative Positions for Childbirth—Part II: Second Stage of Labor," *Journal of Nurse-Midwifery,* vol. 25, no. 5, pp. 13–18.
17. Described in letter to authors, August 8, 1989. Study results were being prepared for publication at that time.
18. Gayle Peterson and Lewis Mehl, *Pregnancy as Healing,* vol. I (Berkeley, California: Mindbody Press, 1984), p. 23.

19. Ibid., p. 22.
20. Ibid., p. 73.
21. Ibid., p. 7.
22. Ibid., p. 97.
23. Ibid., p. 30.

PART FOUR: COMPENSATING FOR THE LOSS

UNMOTHERED MOTHERS

1. Hester Eisenstein, *Contemporary Feminist Thought* (London: Unwin Paperbacks, 1984), p. 69.
2. Ibid.
3. Jean Harley Guilleman and Linda Lytle Holmstrom, "The Business of Childbirth." *Society* (July/August 1986), vol. 23., no. 5, p. 49.
4. The Boston Women's Health Book Collective, *Our Bodies, Our Selves,* Preface to 1973 ed. in the 1976 (2nd) ed. (New York: Simon and Schuster, 1976), p. 13.
5. Ibid., p. 267.
6. Ibid.
7. Grantly Dick-Read, *Childbirth Without Fear,* rev. ed. (New York: Harper & Row, 1984), p. 119.
8. Fernand Lamaze, *Painless Childbirth* (London: Burke, 1958), p. 29.
9. Ibid.
10. Ibid., p. 76.
11. Ibid.
12. Ibid., p. 171.
13. Marjorie Karmel, *Thank You, Dr. Lamaze: A Mother's Experiences in Painless Childbirth,* Dolphin Books ed. (Garden City, New York: Dolphin Books/Doubleday, 1965), p. 45.
14. Irwin Chabon, *Awake and Aware* (New York: Delacorte Press, 1966), p. 124.
15. Ibid., p. 108.
16. Boston Women's Health Collective, *Our Bodies, Our Selves,* 1976 ed., pp. 289–94.
17. Mona Behan, "Childbirth Machisma," *Parenting* (April 1988), p. 54.
18. Sheila Kitzinger, *The Experience of Childbirth,* rev. ed. (London: Victor Gollancz, 1972), p. 19.
19. Ibid., p. 22.
20. Robert A. Bradley, *Husband-Coached Childbirth,* rev. ed. (New York: Harper & Row, 1974), p. 12.
21. Kitzinger, *Experience of Childbirth,* p. 23.

22. Ibid., p. 13.
23. Ibid., p. 216.
24. Bradley, *Husband-Coached*, p. 11.
25. Odent, *Birth Reborn*, p. 28.
26. Ibid., p. 113.

THE STING

1. In addition to opening a Birthing Suite (see pages 247–249), Pennsylvania Hospital also has plans for labor/delivery/recovery (LDRs) rooms. The advantage of these rooms is that a woman may expect to stay in her room for her labor, birth, and for a few hours afterward. This concept is being introduced into many hospitals today, either in this form or as LDRPs—which allow a woman to remain in the same room through the postpartum phase of birth (hence the P of LDRP). They are an important advancement in hospital thinking and design. Certainly they invite less interventive births. They do not, however, teach caregivers the skills and attitudes complementary to the noninterventive births, a problem being addressed by some hospitals through staff retraining programs. At Pennsylvania Hospital, they are exploring the possibility of offering residents an elective month of training with midwives.
2. Lamaze, *Painless Childbirth*, p. 171.
3. Copy available from NAACOG Publications, 409 12th Street, S.W., Washington D.C. 20024-2191.
4. ICEA Position Paper: "The Role of the Childbirth Educator and the Scope of Childbirth Education" (May 1986). Available from ICEA, P.O. Box 20048, Minneapolis, Minnesota 55420-0048.

THE GIVING IN BIRTH

1. This birth story is a composite of three stories told to us by men. Each man was as Doug is presented, i.e., not only enthusiastic about telling his story, but garrulous. One of the men was a TV cameraman.

Acknowledgments

IN THIS book we write that there is a natural power that comes to women when they give birth. Because of our respect for this power and the ultimate dignity it confers on the woman who experiences it, we had to think twice about acknowledging our debts. It wouldn't be correct, for example, to say that each woman who experiences the power is, in the usual meaning of the word, notable. After all, women do not will this thing that comes to them; they do not make it happen. On the other hand, it is inappropriate to ignore the women whom we've watched give birth. In spite of the fact that they are not famous, they have experienced a kind of original power, and the itinerary of power, we read in history, is what we must keep track of.

Thus we were led to acknowledge our debt to something born within each woman, a power not of a woman's making, but one that renews each of us when we witness it, one which refreshes humankind each time a woman feels it. If it were not there, this resilient source, we wouldn't have written as we have. If it were not experienced by individual women, we wouldn't have reason to believe that it can be recovered. We are most grateful, therefore, that we have been permitted to see the original nature of birth.

Next we want to thank the people we interviewed, about a hundred women and about fifteen men. Their willingness to talk to us—strangers—about the intimate details of their births convinced us again that women today, said by many to be distanced from birth and motherhood, are vitally interested in figuring out what happened to them. Birth experiences are as deeply carved in women's psyches as ever before.

We are grateful to Charlotte Houde, CNM, the Director of the Nurse-Midwifery Service, Dartmouth-Hitchcock Hospital at Dartmouth College in Hanover, New Hampshire. She not only arranged for us to interview her and her colleagues, but, to our benefit, she critiqued our theories and our writing. Her challenges, substantive and sensitive to the concerns of today's women, forced us to think much more thoroughly about our hypotheses.

In a related vein, we want to thank the many physicians and midwives, all outrageously busy, who granted us interviews. Most of their names and many of their observations appear in the text. We are equally grateful to the childbirth educators who were willing to describe to us the attitudes and concerns of birthing women today.

Penny is indebted to the late Paul Branca, MD, who introduced her to the concept of lesser intervention for newborn resuscitations; to Ruth Schlegel, ICEA-ICCE, whose professional assistance, personal friendship, and passionate concern for the well-being of birthing women have sustained her; to Mark Cooperstein, MD, whose reliable and reassuring support has been a major factor in the successful continuation of her home-birth practice; to Jane Martin, MS, CNM, and Pat Payne, PhD, CNM, whose work in Lancaster County, Pennsylvania, make it possible for every woman there to have birth options; to Holmes Morton, MD, whose work proves the astonishing healing power of science when it is combined with compassion; to those women who have attended births with her—her mother; Dot; Shirley, Sheryl, Ellie, and Molly; and to the women of the VBAC (Vaginal Birth After Cesarean Section) support group, especially Esther Lantz and Fannie Zook.

We benefited from the thoughtful readings of our drafts by our friends Elaine Galen, Suellen Loebach, Shirley Fischer, and Deborah Schoon. Our editor Liza Dawson helped us immeasurably in understanding what concerns professional women as they become mothers. She and her husband, Havis, even had the courtesy to have their first child, Charlie, while we were working on this book. Alice Martell, our literary agent, also obliged by giving birth to her first child while we wrote. Her enthusiasm for her husband, Mike, her pregnancy, her birth, and her baby, Nicholas, inspired us. That she was able, during the same period, to be enthusiastic about our work, made it impossible for us to lose faith.

More personally, Sheryl is deeply indebted to Nancy Nordhoff, founder of Cottages at Hedgebrook Farm, a retreat for women writers on Whidbey Island in Washington State, for inviting Sheryl to be one of its guests and for her willingness to listen to Sheryl talk her way through her ideas. She is grateful to Rich, Penny's husband, because he has never slacked in his support of Sheryl's writing. She feels an inexpressible appreciation of her sons, Chuck and Mike, and now also to Suzé Kirwan, Mike's partner. Indeed, she is grateful to the entire Kirwan family, who not only know what family is all about, but who have generously shared it with her.

Finally, Penny remembers Susie Preston, a personal friend, who portrayed for her what it is to be deeply rooted in life. She thinks of Rich, whose integrity has guided her and whose love has strengthened her.

Index

281

136–137; differences between, 180–184; hostility of birth reformers and midwives toward, 83; and medical malpractice crisis, 141–145; need for control, 169–170; productivity measures, 140; women's attitudes toward, 109–110
Pithiviers, France, birth at, 42–46, 47–48, 229, 267n
Pitocin, 33, 86, 103, 156–157
Placenta: and delayed cutting of umbilical cord, 43; manual extraction of, 78; praevia, 151
Platt, Dr. Frederick, 137
Poor women: and benefits of midwifery, 81, 82; causes of maternal death, 72
Postpartum depression, 170, 274n
Postpartum hemorrhage, 74, 151, 169
Postpartum infection. See Childbed fever.
Potter, Judy, 212
Power of parenthood: nature of, 32–46; vulnerability of, 20–21, 24–25
Power of women, 115; and birthing energy, 19–21, 58–59; and control by physician, 163; and drugs during labor, 56; loss of, 99; and medicalized birth, 10–11, 199–200; Twilight Sleep and, 12, 95–98
Pregnancy: attitudes of liberated women toward, 209–212; changing caregiver during, 239–240; emotional change during, 153; health during, 81–82; in nineteenth century, 71; tests during, 129, 159–161; and women residents, 177–179
Pregnancy as Healing (Mehl and Peterson), 190–191, 197
Premature infants, touching and, 149
Prenatal care, 128, 82–83; and antepartal complications, 151; fragmentation of, 169; holistic, 190–194; at Pithiviers, 229; and preparation for hospital environment, 43–44; textbook instruction on, 129
Prenatal clinics, 81–82
"Primigravid labor: A graphicostatistical analysis" (Friedman), 150
Professional women. See Career women.
Psychological factors. See Emotional factors.
Public opinion of midwifery, 82–84
Pushing phase of labor, 19, 43

Rebirthing, 124–125
Reddy, Helen, 100, 223
Reich, Eva, 123–124, 125, 126
Religious tradition, labor pain and, 74
Research on birthing, 184–188
Residency of obstetricians, 136–138; and women obstetricians, 177–180

Rich, Adrienne, 108–109
Roberts, Joyce, 188
Roselle, Dr. Amy, 133, 137–138, 140–141, 142, 176
Rosen, Dr. Mortimer, 143
Rothman, Barbara Katz, 160

Sagan, Leonard, 148–149
Savage, Dr. Wendy, 166–174, 184, 193
Savage Enquiry, A: Who Controls Childbirth? (Savage), 167, 172–174
Scientific method: and attitudes toward birth as dangerous, 85–88; and loss of physician-patient communication, 137; and research by midwives, 185–186
Scully, Diana, 134–135, 136, 139
Seigel, Dr. Bernie, 138
Seitchik, Dr. Joseph, 131
Self-control, birth and, 216–219, 227–228; and labor pain, 223–224, 240–241; and Lamaze method, 226–227
Sex education, 101
Sexism: and attitudes toward birthing, 21, 77–78; and medicalized birth, 261
Sex roles, and Amish births, 200–207
Shave. See Perineal shave.
Shearer, Beth, 239, 240
Shearer, Madeleine, 185–186
Shiers, Ruth, 63
Shower. See Bath or shower.
Shumaker, May, 239
Silent Knife (Cohen and Estner), 109
Simchack, Margery, 238
Sinclair, Connie, 64
Smoking, 128
Social Transformation of American Medicine, The (Starr), 76
Sommers, Lisa, 186, 190
Sorger, Dr. Leo, 181–182
Spinals, 98, 102
St. Joseph's Hospital, Lancaster, PA, 234
Starr, Paul, 76
Stevenson, Dr. John, 54
Strong Memorial Hospital, Rochester, NY, 134, 182
Szutowitz, Dr. Mike, 180–181

Tentative Pregnancy (Rothman), 160
Tests, administered by midwives and obstetricians compared, 159–161
Textbooks on obstetrics, 129–130, 150–152, 153
Thank You, Dr. Lamaze (Karmel), 222